Praise for
Understanding Peyronie's Disease

*Peyronie's disease can be an emotionally crippling condition.
Its effects go far beyond the physical problems faced by
a man and his partner. The absence of reliable, accurate,
and credible information for men with Peyronie's disease
has only worsened the situation. But now,
Dr. Levine's book changes that.*

John P. Mulhall, M.D., Director of Sexual Medicine
Memorial Sloan Kettering Cancer Center
Weill Cornell Medical Center

*This book is complete, accurate, and patient-friendly.
It is an excellent resource for men with Peyronie's disease
and their partners.*

Culley Carson, M.D., Chief of Urology
University of North Carolina School of Medicine
Rhodes Distinguished Professor

*I highly recommend this informative book for all men
and their partners. It's the first consumer book to shed light
on this health problem. It is comprehensive, yet easy
to understand. It answers questions and quells the fear
of those who suffer in silence.*

Stan Hardin, President and Co-Founder
Association of Peyronie's Disease Advocates

Understanding
Peyronie's
Disease

A Treatment Guide for Curvature of the Penis

Laurence A. Levine, M.D.

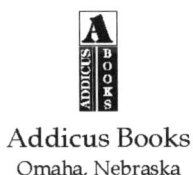

Addicus Books
Omaha, Nebraska

An Addicus Nonfiction Book

ISBN 978-1-886039-85-8

Cover design by Peri Polon-Gabriel

Illustrations by Kristen W. Marzejon, Jack Kusler

Interior design by Linda Dageforde

This book is not intended to serve as a substitute for a physician. Nor is it the author's intent to give medical advice contrary to that of an attending physician.

Library of Congress Cataloging-in-Publication Data

Levine, Laurence A.
  Understanding Peyronie's disease : a treatment guide for curvature of the penis / Laurence A. Levine ;
[illustrations by Kristen W. Marzejon].
      p. Cm.
  "An Addicus nonfiction book"—T.p. Verso.
  Includes index.
1. Penile induration. I. Title.

RC896.L48 2007
616.6'5—dc22   2007014765

Addicus Books, Inc.
P.O. Box 45327
Omaha, Nebraska 68145
www.AddicusBooks.com
Printed in the United States of America
10 9 8 7 6 5 4 3 2 1

Contents

Acknowledgments

I would like to express my gratitude to Linda, Jenna, Sasha, and Reilly Levine for their support of my work in Peyronie's disease. I would also like to thank the Board of Directors of the Association of Peyronie's Disease Advocates, including Marti McKnown, Stan Hardin, and John Mullhall, M.D., for allowing me to participate with them in providing the most reliable source for information about Peyronie's disease available on the Internet and for their support in the development of this patient's guide to Peyronie's disease. I would also like to acknowledge and express my appreciation to the staff at Urology Specialists in Chicago and to Larry Jackel, Rod Colvin of Addicus Books, and Frances Sharpe for their guidance, which helped make this book possible.

Introduction

As a urologist for more than twenty years, I've treated thousands of men with Peyronie's disease and have come to understand the emotional distress, physical pain, and sexual problems this disease can cause. Many of the men I see in my practice complain that they have trouble finding information about Peyronie's disease, its underlying causes, and its treatment. The lack of available, easy-to-understand, accurate information prompted me to write this book. It is intended as a guide for men with Peyronie's disease and their partners or family members who want to learn more about this disabling disorder. I hope that all your questions will be answered within the pages of this book, but it's likely that there will be gaps, which may be addressed by your personal physician. The spirit of this book is to provide useful, accurate, and current information on Peyronie's disease. It should not be considered a substitute for an evaluation by a physician. The opinions expressed are those of the author and may differ from other experts.

Part I

Peyronie's Disease:
An Overview

1

Defining Peyronie's Disease

Whether you have already been diagnosed with *Peyronie's disease* (PD) or think you might have it, you know that the disorder can take a physical and emotional toll. Since the disease affects a very personal and sensitive part of your body—the penis—you may find it difficult to or embarrassing to seek help from your primary care physician or a urologist. As a result, you may, like many other men, suffer in silence and never get a clear understanding of the disease.

Getting accurate information about Peyronie's disease and how it can affect you physically, psychologically, and sexually is the first step to improving your situation. And knowing where to go for help can lead you to the road to recovery.

1. How did Peyronie's disease get its name?

Peyronie's disease was named after François Gigot de la Peyronie, who held the title of First Surgeon to King Louis XIV of France and first wrote about the ailment in 1743. In his classic paper to the medical community, de la Peyronie reported on three men who had an unusual scarring of the penis, which caused deformity. He described the use of special waters coming from a renowned spa in the French town of Barèges to remedy this scar formation; his belief that the disorder was caused by sexually transmitted disease was inaccurate.

2.   What is the medical definition of Peyronie's disease?

Peyronie's disease is considered "a wound-healing disorder." This means that injury or damage to the penile tissues, particularly within the outer penile tissues, activates a scarring process that goes well beyond the normal scarring process.

This excessive scarring can cause painful erections, a curvature of the erect penis, and other penile deformities. In some cases, these symptoms can make it difficult, or even impossible, to engage in sexual intercourse.

3.   What are the symptoms of Peyronie's Disease?

Not every man will have the same onset of symptoms. The PD may develop slowly over time, or the symptoms may develop rapidly. Symptoms may include:

- Hardened scar tissue in the penis
- Pain during erections
- Curvature or bend in the penis when erect
- Narrowing of the diameter of the penis when erect
- Shortening of the erect penis
- Erectile dysfunction

The scarring may occur on the top or bottom of the penis; it can also occur on both sides of the penis.

4.   What kind of penile deformities does Peyronie's disease cause?

There are a variety of penile deformities that can occur as a result of Peyronie's disease, including curvature, indentation, narrowing, hinging, hourglass deformity, and loss of length. The length, location,

Male Reproductive System

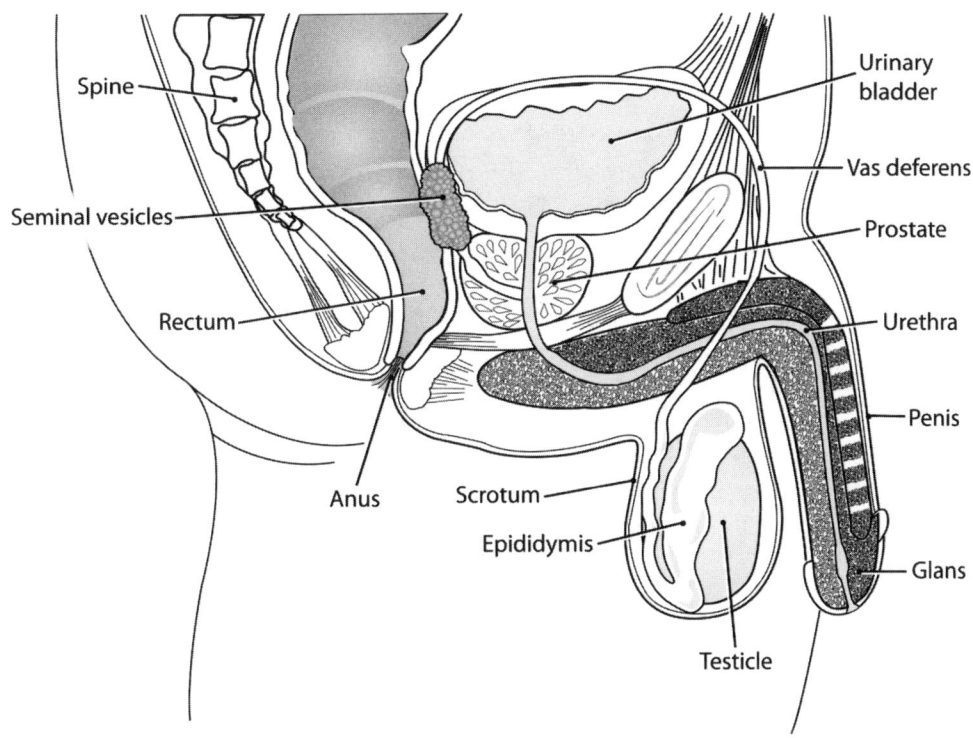

Labels: Spine, Seminal vesicles, Rectum, Anus, Scrotum, Epididymis, Testicle, Urinary bladder, Vas deferens, Prostate, Urethra, Penis, Glans

and orientation of the scar may have an effect on the type of deformity that occurs.

Penile curvature is the most common deformity and most often occurs in an upward direction. However, curvature can also occur in a downward direction or in a lateral direction, meaning the penis curves to one side or the other. Curvature can range from mild to severe. Indentation can occur anywhere on the penis and may lead to narrowing, which means that the shaft loses some of its diameter.

When indentations are severe, it can lead to *hinging*, in which the penis buckles or folds at the point of the indentation. Hinging can also occur when the penis takes on the shape of an hourglass due to a narrowing of the shaft. In this case, the penis will tend to fold or buckle in the narrowed area; this is known as an *hourglass deformity*. Shortening is a common problem and can be the most devastating emotionally. The shortening is typically in the one- to two-inch range, but some men may experience as much as four inches of shortening.

5. Do all patients with Peyronie's disease end up with the same deformity and side effects?

No. The way Peyronie's disease affects each man is highly individual. For instance, some men will develop a large scar but will have very little curvature; others will have what would seem to be very little scar tissue but will have severe curvature with indentation. In addition, up to 30 percent will develop calcification or bone in their scar. Shortening of the penis is common, and the loss of length tends to be due to the extent of scar tissue throughout the shaft of the penis. This is again reflective of the individual nature and behavior of the scarring process. There is also individual variability as to how rapidly the deformity develops as well as how long it takes for the scar to stop growing.

6. What is a Peyronie's plaque?

The scar that forms as a result of this wound-healing disorder is called a *plaque*. This is actually a misnomer, or an incorrect term. Plaque is commonly associated with coronary heart disease and is a mixture of fatty substances, cholesterol, and other substances that become deposited in the inner lining of the arteries. You may worry that having a Peyronie's plaque means you may be at higher risk for having or developing heart disease, but those worries are unfounded. The Peyronie's scar does not contain the same components as cholesterol-containing plaque. In fact, analysis of the Peyronie's tissue shows that it is basically a scar. For the purposes of this book, the terms *scar* and *plaque* will be used interchangeably.

7.   How does the scar cause penile curvature?

Scar tissue that develops on the top of the penis will cause the penis to bend upward. Scarring on the underside of the penis will cause it to bend downward. To better understand this, consider this balloon analogy. If you place a piece of tape on top of the mid-portion of a balloon and then inflate it, the balloon will expand but not in the area that's taped. This results in an upward curvature in the balloon. This is what happens to the penis when excessive scar tissue is present. During an erection, the penis expands except where the scar tissue is located, resulting in curvature or other deformities.

8.   What is the scar made of?

The plaque/scar of Peyronie's disease is in essence like any other scar and has multiple components. The two main components of a typical scar are the proteins *collagen* and *elastin*, the latter of which provides elasticity to tissues. A Peyronie's plaque is also made up of collagen and elastin, however, there is a much greater abundance of collagen than in a typical scar. In addition, both the collagen and elastin in a Peyronie's plaque are disordered, meaning that they do not behave the way they normally would in a typical scar.

Another component that is found in typical scars is *collagenase*, an enzyme that is released at the end of the normal scar-formation process. It breaks down the scar and remodels it down to the smallest possible piece of scar that will hold the tissues together. In the Peyronie's plaque, there is a low or nonexistent level of collagenase, which may explain why the plaque does not go away with time.

9.   Does the size of the plaque affect the degree of deformity?

The size of the plaque does not necessarily correlate to the severity of the deformity. In fact, some men have large plaques but very little curvature. These men may experience loss of shaft length though. Other men who have smaller plaques may have more pronounced curvature.

A Typical Peyronie's Plaque

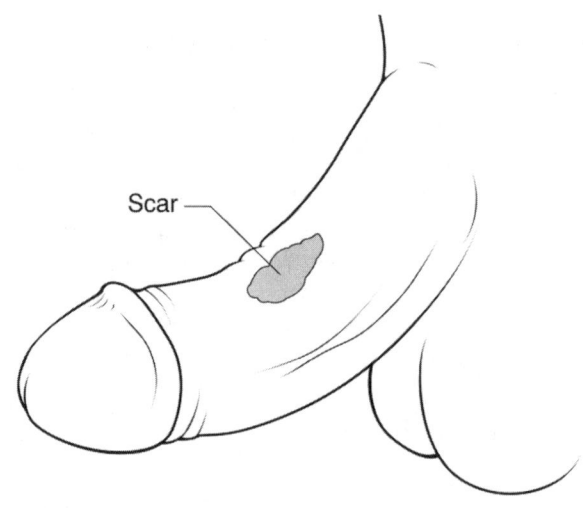

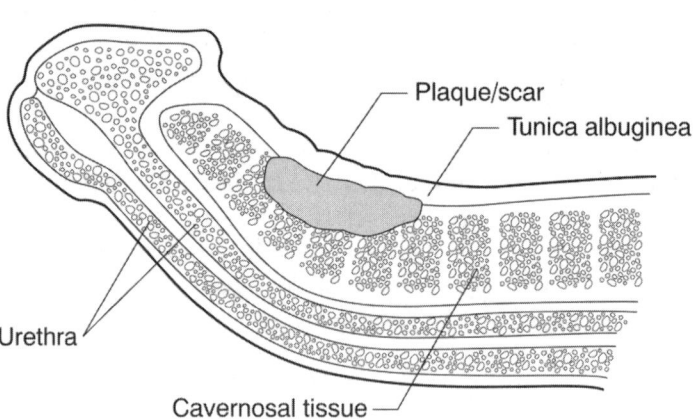

The top illustration shows the exterior of an erect penis with mild Peyronie's disease; the scar tissue is most commonly on the top side of the penis. The lower illustration is an internal view, showing the scar tissue, which is within the penis outer jacket, called the tunica albuginea.

Some experts believe that they can predict the curvature by the length of the plaque. However, this rarely works, as men with extensive plaques on one side of the penis may also have involvement on the opposite side, which may result in counterbalancing the tethering effect of the plaque and thereby reducing the amount of curvature.

10. What kind of changes in the scar can I expect to see with time?

The scar can change in many ways, depending on the individual. It may thicken and spread, it may remain the same size, or in some cases, it may actually get smaller. It is not uncommon to find men who have mild Peyronie's disease who initially reported a nodule in the penis that gradually changed into a long, narrow cord extending sometimes from the head of the penis down into the base. This cord-like thickening process may be an indication of enlargement of the penile *septum*, which is the wall between the two erectile cylinders within the penis. The septum is where the bulk of the pressure is directed during sex. As a result of intercourse, gradual thickening of the septum can occur. Thickening of the septum may also occur as a result of the aging process. In the susceptible man, trauma during intercourse may trigger more aggressive Peyronie's disease with a new lump and further deformity.

Studies have suggested that during the active phase, 50 percent of patients will have worsening of their deformity, around 40 percent will stay the same, and less than 10 percent will have spontaneous resolution of curvature.

11. Do some men develop bone within their plaques?

Reports suggest that anywhere from 12 to 30 percent of men with Peyronie's disease will have varying amounts of calcification within their plaques. Most commonly, it is a stippled or spotty area in which small bits of calcification are scattered around rather than a solid area.

However, in some men, the plaque can form a sizable, irregularly shaped solid bone that can be easily felt through the skin as a hard unbendable structure. This process is known as *dysmorphic calcification*, indicating that it is an abnormal type of bone formation. Currently, researchers believe that this is a variant form of Peyronie's disease since very few men develop the most severe forms of calcification.

12. Is it normal to feel pain from Peyronie's disease?

It's common for pain to be present shortly after an injury to the penis or during the very early stages of Peyronie's disease. During this time, the penis may be painful to the touch, erections may be painful, and attempting intercourse may be painful. The pain associated with Peyronie's disease is due to the inflammation and swelling that occurs within the tissues. This aggravates the pain receptors within the nerves of the penis. Stretching the penis, which occurs with erection, or placing any pressure on the erect penis, can activate the nerves and cause pain. The pain almost always goes away completely within several weeks to a few months.

The simplest treatment to ease the pain associated with Peyronie's disease is to take over-the-counter, nonsteroidal anti-inflammatory medications, such as ibuprofen and naproxen. In rare cases when pain is severe, your physician may give you a prescription for narcotic pain relievers, commonly known as painkillers. Prescription pain pills may be habit-forming and are associated with certain side effects, including drowsiness and a loss of mental alertness. On the other hand, painkillers may be used less frequently and cause less harm to the stomach lining than ibuprofen and naproxen.

There are additional treatments available for pain. Two types of treatment will be covered later in this book; they are injection therapy, in which drugs are injected into the scar tissue, and *electromotive drug administration (EMDA)*, in which electricity is used to deliver drugs

Peyronie's Plaques

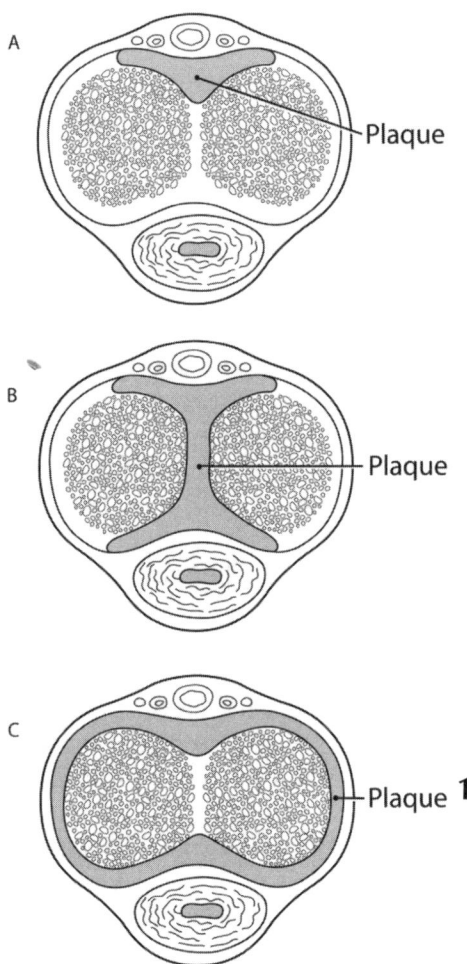

A. The plaque (scar) is on the top side of the penis, causing an upward curve. B. The plaque resembles as "I-beam," and causes narrowing and shortening, but no curvature. C. The plaque surrounds the cylindrical tissue in the penis; this will cause the erect penis to have an hour-glass shape.

through the skin to the scar tissue. These treatments may diminish the local inflammation that causes the pain.

Studies have shown that these treatments can rapidly and permanently resolve the pain. There is also some evidence that pain resolution can be accelerated with shockwave therapy. This is a noninvasive therapy that directs a shock-wave, typically generated by a spark plug, to pass through the skin and focus on the plaque within the penis. However, shock-wave therapy can be expensive and it's probably best to use less costly treatments if you're simply trying to treat pain.

13. What causes Peyronie's disease?

To date, there are no clear-cut answers. However, it has been recognized for some time that Peyronie's disease tends to run in families, suggesting a familial association. There is also likely some underlying genetic abnormality that predisposes a man to be unable to heal injuries to the penis in a normal fashion. In the past, it was thought that Peyronie's disease might be caused by an *autoimmune* disease or by an infection, but these causes have not been confirmed. Likewise, at this time, it appears that PD does not occur due to the use of any medications.

In the past decade, there has been increased interest among researchers worldwide to try to understand what causes PD. Thanks to this increased interest, we should gain a better understanding of what is responsible for this penile scar formation.

14. How does Peyronie's disease develop?

Peyronie's disease typically develops in two stages: acute and stable. During the acute phase, which typically follows injury or trauma to the penis, it's common to experience a sensation of pain in the penis. The pain may be felt anywhere within the penis, but is often felt in the head, or *glans*, of the penis. You may feel pain when touching the penis or with an erection. The pain may worsen when attempting penetration during sexual activity. During this stage, you may notice a palpable lump or nodule on the penis but may not have any curvature. Either at this time or shortly thereafter, depending upon the aggressiveness of the plaque formation, the deformity occurs with curvature, shortening, and/or indentation. Once the pain subsides and the deformity stops changing for a period of time, the disease is considered to be in the stable stage.

There have been very few studies on the *natural history* of PD, meaning what happens if you do nothing to have the disorder treated. As mentioned earlier, it is believed that it will dissipate in about 10 percent of men; however, if the deformity completely resolves with disappearance of the scar tissue, it is unlikely that it was Peyronie's disease and was probably just a slow-healing wound within the penis. For the most part, if curvature is to improve spontaneously, it tends to occur within the first one to two years from the onset of the disease.

15. Does Peyronie's disease tend to develop suddenly or gradually?

The deforming process is most often gradual and can take months to develop. However, there is no routine time frame for the development of Peyronie's disease, and in some cases, the deforming process can happen very quickly, as in a matter of weeks. In some men, the scarring process can be so aggressive that it would seem the deformity occurs "overnight." The majority of men will initially experience pain and a palpable nodule followed sometime later by curvature or some other penile deformity. The disease stabilizes anywhere from one to eighteen months after the curvature is noted.

16. If Peyronie's disease develops quickly, does that mean that the curvature will be more severe?

It is not necessarily the case that if you experience sudden and aggressive scarring, you will end up with a severely deformed penis. In fact, the rate at which Peyronie's disease develops does not appear to have much effect on the severity of the deformity.

17. When do I know that the deformity associated with Peyronie's disease has stopped progressing?

You will know that the Peyronie's process has stabilized and that it is unlikely that the deformity will get worse when there is no pain with the development of an erection and when the plaque and deformity have not changed for at least four to six months. These time periods have not been universally agreed upon and have been mostly based upon physician experience and the published literature in the medical journals. In some men, stabilization can be reached within several months, but in others, it may take up to eighteen months from the time of onset.

18. Can I develop Peyronie's disease without ever having injured my penis?

The current medical thinking is that Peyronie's disease does result from an injury to the penis. It is not known scientifically whether it may develop without an injury. The injury may occur to either an erect or flaccid penis.

Note: Up to 60 percent of the men I see in my practice are not aware of any injury that may have activated the Peyronie's disease. The other 40 percent recall that following the injury there was a period of pain, a palpable lump, and then deformity.

19. Can Peyronie's disease occur later...perhaps a year after injury to the penis?

The straightforward answer to this question is "Yes." That is because it may be that the initial injury did not actually trigger the Peyronie's, but a subsequent silent injury may have set the abnormal scarring process in motion.

20. What are the most common triggering events that cause the scarring associated with Peyronie's disease?

The current thinking is that Peyronie's disease develops most commonly following trauma to the erect penis during sexual activity. However, multiple studies have shown that men may develop Peyronie's disease after an injury to the *flaccid* penis, or they may not recall any injury at all.

Trauma during sexual activity may be due to high pressures that occur within the tissues of the penis during intercourse and which may cause microfractures that activate the abnormal wound-healing process. Pressure in the penis is measured in millimeters of mercury (mm Hg), the same way blood pressure is measured. Internal pressures in the flaccid penis measure 5-10 mm Hg. In the erect state, the penis has an internal pressure of approximately 70-90 mm Hg. However, during sexual activity, if the penis were to become compressed against the vaginal tissues or be thrust against a nonreceptive area such as a thigh or buttock, then pressures can exceed 800 mm Hg. This kind of pressure could easily snap a bone and is why it is believed that the penis is most commonly injured in the erect state during intercourse.

Note: Interestingly, the majority of my patients do not recall any event where they may have injured the penis. Those who do remember report what has come to be known as "rodeo sex," in which the female partner is on top. This puts the penis at greater risk for a mis-thrust or very high pressures. Up to 10 percent of my PD patients recall trauma to the flaccid penis that has occurred as the result of a motor vehicle accident or some other direct trauma to the penis that has occurred during physical exercise or randomly during the course of a day. The key is that the abnormal wound-healing process may be activated even if you don't remember experiencing an injury or trauma to the penis.

21. Will every man develop Peyronie's disease following an injury to the penis?

No. In fact, nearly every man injures his penis at some point during his lifetime. The vast majority of them will simply heal normally from the injury. There may be pain, but it will subside and there will be no lasting effects due to the injury. It's only in certain men that the abnormal scarring process is activated and Peyronie's disease develops.

22. Is Peyronie's disease a genetic disorder that runs in families?

It is unclear whether Peyronie's disease is a genetic disorder, but it does appear to run in families. Multiple studies have shown irregularities in the chromosomes in the tissues of men with Peyronie's disease. Also noted is chromosomal instability, which means that chromosomes may be prone to change from normal behavior to abnormal behavior in damaged penile tissue. It will take some time to work out the details of this process, but there is no doubt that Peyronie's disease appears to be a familial disorder. If one member of a family has Peyronie's disease, his brothers, father, or sons may be at higher risk for developing it, too. Exactly how much higher the risk is has not been determined.

23. If I have PD, should I talk to my brothers or sons about the disorder?

It's a good idea to discuss the problem with your brothers or sons. It's understandable that sharing your personal medical information may be difficult, particularly when it involves sexual problems. However, as our society matures and men become more comfortable talking about these issues, it may be easier to bring up this difficult topic with other members of the family.

If you are considering talking to your adolescent or older sons regarding Peyronie's disease, inform them that a deformity of the penis may occur as a result of injury during sex. Emphasize that they should simply be careful during sexual activity and, if possible, avoid bending the erect penis excessively. This may be especially good advice for the young man who may be performing vigorous or excessive masturbation.

Lastly, it may be useful to discuss Peyronie's disease with other male family members so that if they develop a painful lump in the penis—with or without deformity—they'll know that it should be evaluated by a doctor as soon as possible. It is not likely that this type of discussion will prevent Peyronie's disease from occurring, but it may encourage pursuit of an evaluation with a physician, which may help prevent progression of the scar and deformity.

24. If I have a family history of Peyronie's disease, can I take preventative measures?

If you know that Peyronie's disease runs in your family, you should realize that you are at an increased risk of developing this problem as you get older. There is no clear way to avoid Peyronie's disease except for avoiding trauma during sex, which appears to be the most common triggering event activating this abnormal scarring process. It's best to avoid unusual positions or pressures on the penis, which may be more apt to occur when your sexual partner is on top.

25. Can I determine whether I am susceptible to developing Peyronie's disease?

Unfortunately, there is no clear answer to this question at this time. To date, there are no biological markers, blood tests, or any other indicators of Peyronie's disease. However, two things that may increase your risk include a family history of the disease or having a condition called *Dupuytren's contracture*, a scarring disorder involving the palm and surface of the hand; this contracture has a similar genetic makeup to the scarring that occurs in PD. How so? Dupuytren's contracture is marked by a thickening and shrinking of the layer of flesh just under the skin of the palm, which leads to the curvature of one or more of the fingers and an inability to straighten them. The condition usually creates a thick scar that feels like a nodule or lump within the palm of the hand.

What is distinctive is that up to 20 percent of men who have a Dupuytren's contracture in one or both hands also later developed Peyronie's disease. This means that if those men with Dupuytren's contractures experience a penile injury, it may result in excessive scarring in the penis.

26. Do sexually transmitted diseases cause PD?

Many men commonly ask this question. However, there is no evidence that Peyronie's disease is due to any type of sexually transmitted disease (STD) or any other type of infection, including from bacterial, viral, or fungal organisms.

27. Can medical conditions, such as hypertension and diabetes, increase the risk of Peyronie's disease?

Hypertension, or high blood pressure, may have an indirect link to Peyronie's disease. Hypertension has been associated with *erectile dysfunction* (ED) since it causes progressive injury to the blood vessels within the penis, reducing the ability of those vessels to dilate in response to a sexual stimulus. When you have compromised erections, you can injure your penis while trying to have intercourse with a soft erection. It may be that the buckling that occurs with a less rigid penis results in microtrauma in the penis, which could activate the Peyronie's process. This type of injury is similar to a metal-fatigue fracture that happens from bending a piece of soft metal back and forth on multiple occasions until the metal fractures.

Large-scale studies of patients with Peyronie's disease have demonstrated that there appears to be a higher-than-expected rate of high blood pressure, elevated cholesterol, and diabetes in patients with Peyronie's disease. According to these studies, anywhere from 12 to 40 percent of patients may have one or more of these conditions. In the past, it was believed that these medical problems resulted in decreased blood flow to the penis. They are recognized as the primary risk factors for erectile dysfunction.

It is now being suggested that these disorders may be independent risk factors for Peyronie's disease, which means that if you have high blood pressure, elevated cholesterol, and/or diabetes, you may be at a higher risk for Peyronie's disease even without the presence of erectile dysfunction. Why these diseases result in PD remains unknown at this time, but it may be the associated erectile dysfunction that makes the penis more susceptible to injury.

28. Is stress a possible trigger for Peyronie's disease?

Stress is a contributing factor to many disorders, and it may play a role in PD as well. It is unlikely that stress would activate the Peyronie's process directly, but stress may result in diminished rigidity in the erect penis. Engaging in intercourse with a soft erection increases the likelihood of injury, which would then activate the Peyronie's process in a susceptible individual. As medicine advances, and we know more about the psychodynamic aspects of stress, we may find that anxiety and stress actually do have physiological responses that can activate the scarring process. At this time, however, it is more likely to be coincidental or due to a traumatic event that happened with a less rigid erection during a stressful period in your life.

29. Does masturbation cause Peyronie's disease?

Masturbation doesn't cause PD, however, an injury to the erect penis during masturbation could activate the disease in the susceptible individual. This type of injury is most apt to occur if the penis has excessive pressures being placed on it, causing it to bend excessively in one direction or another. This can cause microtrauma within the penis, which can activate the abnormal wound-healing process associated with Peyronie's disease. Although it is rare, PD has been reported in teenagers who may have activated it through vigorous masturbation.

Many younger men who have developed Peyronie's disease indicate that the only time when they may have injured their penis would have been during vigorous masturbation during which the penis may be bent excessively or otherwise traumatized. Typically this involves momentary pain, which may result in loss of the erection, but then the Peyronie's process may occur in the future.

30. What is jelquing, and does it cause Peyronie's disease?

Jelquing is the act of grabbing the erect penis and pushing down in a vigorous way in effort to prolong ejaculation, to get rid of an unwanted erection, or to stretch the length of the penis. Interestingly, a published report from Iran, where jelquing is used frequently to reduce an unwanted erection or to enhance better control over ejaculation, showed that the risk of developing Peyronie's disease was no higher in this population than in the general population.

Note: In my opinion, this report neither suggests that jelquing is a good thing to do, nor does it dispel the concept that trauma may activate Peyronie's disease. On the other hand, it may suggest that the young men evaluated in this study were not susceptible to Peyronie's disease and therefore the trauma would not result in scarring. It is my opinion that jelquing increases the potential for development of Peyronie's disease in the susceptible individual and is not recommended.

31. Can surgery for prostate cancer trigger Peyronie's disease?

Up to 10 percent of men who have undergone a specific surgical treatment for prostate cancer have reported developing Peyronie's disease. The treatment in question is called a *radical retropubic prostatectomy* and involves removal of the prostate. The reason for this correlation with PD remains unclear, but the prostate is in very close proximity to the penis, and surgery in this area may activate the disordered wound-healing process. It is highly unlikely that the Peyronie's disease process is activated by the urinary catheter used during the surgical procedure. Any trauma resulting from the use of a urinary catheter would typically result in a downward or ventral curvature, and most of the patients who develop PD after radical prostate surgery will develop an upward or lateral curvature.

32. Could a cystoscopy be a factor in developing PD?

A *cystoscopy* is a procedure in which a slender rigid tube called a *cystoscope* is inserted into the *urethra* in order to view it and the bladder. It is unlikely that this procedure or any type of urethral manipulation would trigger Peyronie's disease. However, a downward bend to the penis would suggest that urethral trauma may have activated some inflammation and scarring on the undersurface of the penis, causing the downward curve. The majority of men who have Peyronie's disease have either an upward or lateral curve. If you have an upward or lateral curve, it is highly unlikely that it was due to any type of urethral manipulation, including cystoscopy.

33. How common is Peyronie's disease?

It's hard to determine just how common Peyronie's disease is. Studies from the 1980s showed that less than 1 percent of men reported having PD. However, those studies only included men who went to the hospital to seek treatment for their symptoms. Newer studies show that while performing routine screening exams for prostate cancer, doctors noted PD in approximately 10 percent of their male patients. Some men who have this condition choose not to seek treatment from a medical professional. This may be for a variety of reasons. For instance, symptoms may be so mild that PD doesn't interfere with their daily routines or sexual activity, or perhaps they're too embarrassed to talk to their doctor about it. Because of this, the percentage of men who have Peyronie's disease may actually be much higher than expected.

34. Who gets Peyronie's disease?

Medical studies show that Peyronie's disease occurs most often in men in their mid-fifties. However, it can also occur in teenagers as well as in men in their eighties. Peyronie's disease is primarily seen in Caucasian men, although does not discriminate, and can occur in men of any race or ethnicity. It may seem to be more prevalent in Caucasian men because they may seek treatment more often than men of other ethnic backgrounds.

Note: In my practice, I have seen African-American, Hispanic, East Indian, American Indian and Asian men—including Chinese, Japanese, and Korean men—with PD.

35. Why does PD occur most often in men who are in their fifties?

Virtually all of the published studies on Peyronie's disease have found that the average age of men who develop Peyronie's disease tends to be in the early to mid-fifties. This may be because natural aging causes changes, such as reduced rigidity, in the penis. This may subject the penis to a greater risk of injury, which activates the underlying Peyronie's disease. It is also possible that PD is simply an age-related phenomenon that becomes activated by an abnormal response to a penile injury in the fifth decade or beyond. But men of any age can develop Peyronie's disease. In two studies, up to 10 percent of men who reported Peyronie's disease were under the age of forty. These young men with Peyronie's disease are more likely to recall a specific event where the penis was injured.

36. Is there a difference between younger and older men who develop PD as far as outcome?

Young men with Peyronie's disease tend to have better erections following the onset of Peyronie's disease and seem to respond better to all forms of treatment as compared to older men with PD. This is likely because of the better vascular condition of the erectile tissue in younger men, making for better quality rigidity after treatment. It is also presumed that the younger men are more likely to respond better to treatment since the tissues of younger men appear to have the capacity to heal more quickly and completely than in those of older men. Still, there are significant psychological issues that can occur in men of any age that can compromise erectile response and sexual function after developing Peyronie's disease.

37. Do most men adjust psychologically to the changes in their penis?

In most cases, men can adjust psychologically to the changes in the penis due to Peyronie's disease or due to treatment to correct it—even if they're left with a somewhat smaller or slightly crooked penis. Clearly, the goal of treatment is to regain as close to the full, natural penis you had before developing Peyronie's disease, but this is highly unlikely. Therefore the real expectation is to become sexually functional again and to accept the changes that have occurred. It's similar to having to accept the changes that may occur with trauma to the knee or back, which may make you unable to exercise in the same way you did as a young man.

38. Does having Peyronie's disease cause depression among most men?

The problem of depression, anxiety, and loss of self-esteem as a result of Peyronie's disease is now recognized to be quite common. Studies show that 70 to 90 percent of men have significant emotional distress as a result of having PD. This is because of the importance of the penis to a man's sense of masculinity. When the penis changes in a negative way, it can have an overwhelming effect on you.

Anxiety and depression can interfere with your functions in life at all levels, including sexual activity with a partner, family interaction, and activities at work. Peyronie's disease can cause a general negative feeling about yourself that can lead to depression or even to suicidal thoughts, which needs to be treated medically. The key to taking control over the depression is seeking an evaluation to confirm the presence of Peyronie's disease, having the necessary discussions with your physician, and choosing the appropriate treatment. In some cases, taking these actions may be all that is necessary to reduce or eliminate your feelings of depression. However, if this is not enough, and if the effects of the disease are too devastating, then referral to a psychiatrist or sex therapist may be necessary.

39. Can I take antidepressants for the depression that I am experiencing as a result of my Peyronie's disease?

It is not unusual for men with Peyronie's disease to take antidepressant medications to help them get through the adjustment period of having this disorder. There are a variety of antidepressant medications available, and your physician will determine which is most appropriate for you. Wellbutrin may be recommended because it seems to have fewer sexual side effects than other antidepressants. Or, your doctor may prescribe a selective serotonin reuptake inhibitor (SSRI). These drugs help the brain make better use of the neuro-chemical serotonin. When used in low doses, SSRIs may not only help with depressive symptoms but may also delay orgasm, which can reduce premature ejaculation, something that may accompany Peyronie's disease.

If you're feeling depressed about having Peyronie's disease, it's important to remember that there are proven medical and surgical treatments that can improve the situation. You should make an appointment with a urologist rather than try unproven treatments advertised on Web sites.

40. Is evidence that antidepressant drugs, such as Lexapro, may contribute to the cause of PD?

At this point there is no evidence that taking any medication, including the antidepressant medication Lexapro, has any effect on the development of Peyronie's disease. In the past, medical journal articles on Peyronie's disease suggested that various medications may have some effect on the development of the disease. But these articles were typically based on very small numbers of patients. Many men are using a variety of antidepressants at this time, and yet there does not appear to be an increased occurrence of Peyronie's disease in men using these medications.

41. Does penile cancer also produce the plaque-like growths in the penis shaft like Peyronie's disease?

There are rare penile cancers known as *fibrosarcomas* that have a thickened scar-like mass in the shaft of the penis. They tend to occur within the vascular tissue of the penis rather than in the outer jacket where the scarring associated with PD typically occurs. Fibrosarcomas tend to grow whereas Peyronie's plaques may expand but do not tend to grow into the spongy vascular tissue of the penis. There are other types of cancers of the penis which may involve the urethra and may be felt along the undersurface of the penis extending from the penile tip to the base of the penis. If you find a lump within the penis, seek an evaluation either by your primary care physician, or better yet, a urologist. A physical examination by a doctor will hopefully help rule out cancer and determine whether you have PD.

Note: In more than twenty years of seeing patients with Peyronie's disease, I have encountered only one fibrosarcoma and this was in a patient who had a very large mass within the penis that did not resemble Peyronie's disease.

42. Can Peyronie's disease turn into cancer?

No, Peyronie's disease does not develop into cancer. PD is *benign fibrosis*, which simply means a noncancerous scarring process. It's understandable that you might become frightened that a palpable nodule in your penis may be an indication of cancer. Typical of men, this may result in a "bury your head in the sand" response in hopes that it will go away spontaneously rather than seek immediate medical care. Be assured that penile cancer is rare in the United States. Even so, it is advisable for any man who notices a lump or nodule within the penis to be evaluated by a primary care physician or a urologist to rule out cancer or to identify the Peyronie's process and be able to initiate treatment if indicated.

43. As long as I can remember, I have had curvature in my penis when it is erect. Is this Peyronie's disease?

When a man has a lifelong history of penile curvature, it is considered a congenital curvature. This deformity is called *chordee*. Congenital curvature of the penis is not uncommon and can cause an upward, downward, or lateral bend. Curvature can range from mild to severe and may or may not interfere with sexual intercourse. Congenital curvature is not caused by Peyronie's disease.

The exact cause of chordee is not understood, but it is likely due to excessive elasticity on one side of the penis relative to the other. Unlike Peyronie's disease, in which a scar causes restricted expansion, in a young man with chordee, there is excessive elasticity resulting in the deformity. Most men with chordee have a downward curvature. In this circumstance, the elasticity of the tissues on the top side of the penis is greater than on the undersurface, resulting in the downward curvature.

44. I am twenty-two, and my erect penis curves slightly to the left. I feel no pain or lumps during masturbation. Is this Peyronie's disease and should I seek treatment?

It is likely that the slight curvature that you see is a natural curve seen in many men. In fact, a curvature of less than 30 degrees in any direction is considered within the normal range, as it is not likely to interfere with sexual activity. If your curvature interferes with sexual activity, then you should consult with a physician about treatment.

45. I am nineteen, and my penis has a downward bend. I don't feel any scar tissue, and I don't have erection problems;

however, the curve in my penis prevents me from having intercourse. Could I have Peyronie's disease?

This sounds more like chordee, which is not associated with scarring and which typically results in a downward curvature. If the curvature is significantly downward, it can make penetrative sex difficult to impossible and occasionally quite uncomfortable for the female partner. The best approach for you would be to see a urologist who has experience treating congenital curvature with surgical straightening.

46. If I have chordee, can I also develop Peyronie's disease?

Although this is not reported frequently, it can occur. If you have a genetic predisposition to Peyronie's disease and also injure the penis sufficiently, most commonly during intercourse, you could possibly activate underlying Peyronie's disease and make the curvature worse. You would know that Peyronie's disease had occurred if the curvature of the penis got dramatically worse or if there was sudden, marked shortening of the penis. Most men with chordee have a long penis because of the increased elasticity. Therefore the shortening may be due to the scarring process, which is restricting expansion of the penis.

47. I injured my penis during sex. I heard a loud popping sound. Is this what's called a penile fracture? Does this mean I will develop Peyronie's disease?

A penile fracture is a medical emergency that most commonly occurs when the penis is erect during intercourse. In this circumstance, the penis is bent excessively in one direction or another, placing extremely high pressure on the outer jacket of the penis. The outer jacket can only withstand so much stretching before the tissues tear and if the tear is full thickness, this results in what is known as a penile fracture. Men who have experienced a penile fracture frequently recall a loud "popping" sound associated with pain, rapid onset of bruising, loss of erection, swelling, and deformity of the penis.

When this occurs, the best thing to do is to seek emergency attention within the first twenty-four hours following the injury to determine whether the fracture should be repaired right away to reduce the likelihood of subsequent deformity and/or erectile dysfunction. Repairing a fracture is an outpatient procedure that requires anesthesia. During the procedure, the skin of the penis is pulled away to expose the tear, any blood that has pooled in the area is removed, any damaged tissue in the area is removed, and the tear is closed with absorbable sutures.

Most men who undergo surgical repair of a fracture do not develop subsequent Peyronie's disease. This may be because the fracture is full thickness and is not a contained injury, which might be more apt to activate the Peyronie's process. On the other hand, the genetically susceptible man who experiences a penile fracture may also develop Peyronie's disease. These men should be treated like any other man with Peyronie's disease, using the noted medical and/or surgical treatments discussed in other sections.

48. I experienced a penile fracture and did not get immediate care; I then developed deformity and erectile dysfunction. What should I do now?

In this circumstance, evaluation by a urologist with expertise in erectile dysfunction and Peyronie's disease is recommended. A urologist can determine whether the erectile dysfunction and deformity are due to internal scarring within the penile vascular tissue caused by the penile fracture, or whether Peyronie's disease is contributing to the deformity as well. Sometimes, the tearing process results in scarring of the internal vascular tissue preventing blood flow beyond the area of the fracture, thereby destabilizing and softening the penis and potentially resulting in curvature as well.

This condition is best evaluated using ultrasound technology known as *color dynamic duplex ultrasonography*. This is an outpatient procedure that doesn't require anesthesia and typically takes less than one hour to return results, which can yield a good deal of information about what is going on inside the penis and why it is deformed and/or not getting fully erect.

49. I had a piercing in my penis a couple of years ago. After I had the opening for the piercing stretched to 5 mm, a lump and a bend occurred in my penis. Have you heard of this before? Is it coincidental?

Any traumatic event to the penis can activate Peyronie's disease in the susceptible individual. From your question, it is not exactly clear where your piercing is located on the penis, but usually it is in the area of the urethral opening of the penis, which is well out of the area where Peyronie's disease occurs. Therefore, it is more likely that you had a separate, perhaps silent injury to the penis that activated the Peyronie's process. Because of this, it is most likely coincidental and not due to the piercing.

50. Where can I find current, valid, and useful information regarding Peyronie's disease on the Internet?

If you're looking for accurate information about Peyronie's disease on the Internet, visit www.peyroniesassociation.org, which is the site for the Association of Peyronie's Disease Advocates (APDA), or www.peyronies.org, which is sponsored by a urologist with experience in the disease. Both of these sites offer good information about Peyronie's disease, but they cannot accurately diagnose your problem or offer individualized treatment solutions for you. Only a qualified physician can provide you with a diagnosis and the appropriate treatment options for you.

A number of chat rooms and blogs about Peyronie's disease have formed over the years. Some of these Web sites provide an opportunity for men who suffer from PD, or their partners who are suffering with them, to vent, share their experiences, and also offer recommendations about home remedies. Unfortunately, none of these home remedies have been studied, and it is unlikely that they would result in any real improvement to the Peyronie's scarring process.

51. Where are the research laboratories that are currently studying Peyronie's disease?

There are only a few laboratories in the U.S. that are studying Peyronie's disease from a basic science perspective. This means that they are developing techniques to evaluate the actual content and function of the tissue in men with Peyronie's disease. In addition, they are developing animal models of Peyronie's with hopes that this will shed light on its underlying cause and allow development of new treatment options. The premier laboratories studying Peyronie's disease in the U.S. at this time are located at UCLA, University of California San Francisco, Tulane University in New Orleans, Rush University Medical Center in Chicago, and Cornell University Medical Center in New York City.

Researchers are hopeful that as governmental agencies, pharmaceutical companies, and device manufacturers gain more interest in Peyronie's disease, they will contribute to research on the disease. Among the benefits of additional funds for research will be a growing number of scientists who are interested in the disease and therefore more understanding of and treatments for PD.

52. What's a clinical trial and what is involved in a clinical trial for Peyronie's disease?

A clinical trial uses human subjects to test the efficacy of a drug or treatment method. There are many criteria that doctors and scientists use to say that the results of a scientific or clinical study are valid and meaningful. In the case of Peyronie's disease, it has been suggested that this would include studies that evaluate the men completely in terms of their deformity, pretreatment sexual function, pain level, and penile length, as well as assessments of calcification, plaque size, and duration of disease. It would also include studies where the erect deformity can be measured both at the beginning of the study and at the end of treatment so any changes can be documented.

Simply asking a patient whether there has been a positive change following treatment is unfortunately quite flawed. For a number of reasons, patients may give inaccurate answers to questions directed to them by the doctor treating them. Therefore, anonymous and properly evaluated questionnaires are necessary. In addition, what are known as objective measures are obtained. An objective measure is one that can be obtained by different individuals and is both reliable and repeatable. The critical measurements for men with Peyronie's disease are penile length, penile curvature, indentation or narrowing, and overall sexual function and erectile rigidity. These objective measures must be evaluated both before and after treatment.

Having a placebo group would also assist in understanding whether the treatment is truly providing some benefit over just time alone. A placebo is an inert substance used in controlled experiments to test the efficacy of another drug. Doing this type of study has proven to be difficult in men with Peyronie's disease. In part, this is because men are quite distressed about the disease and frequently are not willing to participate in a placebo-controlled trial because they fear they may receive the placebo and therefore no benefit. As doctors and scientists become more educated about designing clinical trials, the hope is that even men who receive a placebo would ultimately have an opportunity to receive the treatment drug. Lastly, the studies must be of adequate size in terms of the number of men participating in the study. The groups of men in the treatment versus the placebo group should be similar in terms of their duration of disease, the nature of their deformity, whether they have or do not have calcification in their plaque, and their overall sexual function.

53. Can a new penis be generated from DNA or stem cell therapy?

There is ongoing research at Bowman Gray Medical Center on a variety of different tissues that may be developed for future transplantation. These include the lining of the urethra, the bladder, and possibly even the corporeal tissues of the penis. A full artificial penis developed in the laboratory has not yet been reported, but may be on the distant horizon.

2

Evaluation of Peyronie's Disease

It's important to seek evaluation by a primary care physician or a urologist as soon as possible if you feel a lump or nodule in your penis, if you have penile curvature or some other deformity, or if you feel pain when touching your penis or when developing an erection. Pursuing an evaluation in the early stage of Peyronie's disease is important. In the early stage of the disease, the scarring process is building rapidly, and treatment can be effective in preventing the condition from getting worse, and in some cases, may even reverse the symptoms.

Another reason to seek medical evaluation as soon as possible is to rule out cancer. Although it is extremely rare, there are unusual cancers of the penis that may mimic a Peyronie's plaque. These tumors are called fibrosarcomas and can be deadly if left to progress. A urologist can evaluate any growths present and, if necessary, perform a biopsy, in which tissues are surgically removed and examined for cancer.

1.   What should I expect from an evaluation for Peyronie's disease?

An evaluation by a urologist who has expertise in Peyronie's disease should take about twenty to thirty minutes. During this evaluation, the doctor should provide you with basic information about Peyronie's disease, including its causes, symptoms, and treatment options—both surgical and nonsurgical. The physician will ask you when you first noticed changes in your penis and whether you recall experiencing any injury or trauma to the penis.

In addition, the doctor will ask whether you have other medical conditions, such as the hand deformity Dupuytren's contracture, or erectile dysfunction, including premature ejaculation or diminished penile sensation. The doctor will also take a thorough medical history to determine whether you are at risk for vascular disease as a result of diabetes, high blood pressure, elevated cholesterol, or smoking. You will likely be asked to give a detailed assessment of your penile deformity in terms of direction of curvature, degree of curvature, shortening, indentation, hinging, or buckling.

The physician should then perform a full physical examination focusing on the penis. Your physician will likely measure the stretched length of your flaccid penis. To do this, the physician will gently pull the penis until it reaches its full extended length. The length of the penis can change with time as Peyronie's disease develops, which is why having a baseline length assessment can be useful. Taking photographs of your penis in the erect state to the physician's office can also be helpful; the photos can show the physician the severity of your problem and help him or her develop appropriate treatment options. If you plan to take photos to your appointment, take the pictures while looking down at the erect penis; also take pictures from the side. Your evaluation may include additional testing.

2. What additional tests may be included in an evaluation?

Your doctor may choose to perform some additional imaging studies of your penis. For instance, a standard x-ray may be taken to ensure that there is no calcification in the plaque. The imaging study most commonly performed is a color dynamic duplex ultrasound. Similar to an ultrasound test that allows a doctor to see inside the uterus of a pregnant woman, a color dynamic duplex ultrasound test allows a physician to see inside the penis. The "duplex" part of the test also allows the doctor to measure blood flow in the penis. This painless procedure is noninvasive and involves placing a jelly-like substance on the penis and then passing a wand on the penis.

A color dynamic duplex ultrasound study is an outpatient procedure that can either be performed in the doctor's office or in the radiology department. Typically an initial scanning of the penis is performed looking for calcification (bone) within the plaque as well as within the vascular tissue. A painless injection of a drug is then given, which causes blood vessel dilation and erection. During the development of the erection, a series of measurements are made to evaluate blood flow in the penis. The goal here is to obtain a full erection, which would indicate satisfactory blood flow. At the same time, penile deformities can be measured. Curvature is measured with a protractor, and irregularities in girth are measured with a string wrapped around the circumference of the penis at various points.

Once the test is complete, the erection usually goes away on its own. However, if the drug-induced erection does not spontaneously reverse, you can expect to receive a second injection, which should reverse or "bust" the erection. These injections have no long-term, negative effects on your penis or your erection. They are short-acting drugs that are quickly metabolized and disappear with no lasting effects. Rarely, men will have a small nodule in the area of injection, which will resolve. These small nodules do not become new Peyronie's plaques.

Your physician may also recommend certain blood tests, including a blood testosterone level. Testosterone is a hormone that affects your sex drive. Once your physician has your full medical history, physical examination, and imaging studies, appropriate treatment options can be discussed.

3. Will my doctor be able to tell me if I'm in the early stage or stable stage of Peyronie's disease?

Based on the information you provide, your doctor should be able to determine which stage of the disease you are in. Peyronie's disease typically evolves from an acute stage—an early stage when the disease is unstable—to a stable stage when deformity remains but has not changed for some time. The acute stage seems to occur shortly after activation by injury or trauma to the penis and is recognized by a penis that is painful to the touch or with an erection. Also during this time, a palpable scar or nodule on the penis may be changing in shape and deformity of the penis—including curvature, indentation, and/or shortening—may be developing. The acute or early phase may last up to six to twelve months.

Stable or late-phase Peyronie's disease is recognized by a deformity, which may include indentation, shortening, or curvature and a scar that has not changed for six to nine months. The pain experienced when touching the penis, with an erection, or during intercourse typically has disappeared in stable or late-stage disease. Some men may have such advanced curvature that the stretching of the penis during attempts to have intercourse may activate pain. This is different from the inflammatory pain associated with early or acute disease.

4. Is there a better prognosis if I have no pain at the onset of this disease?

Studies show that thirty to forty percent of men who develop Peyronie's disease experience no pain with erection or during attempts at intercourse. Even so, they can still develop a severe deformity similar to those who do experience pain at the beginning of the disease process. Therefore, having no pain at the onset of PD doesn't mean you'll have a better prognosis with respect to long-term outcome. However, it is certainly more comfortable if you are pain-free as the pain associated with PD can be quite disturbing.

5. I have had Peyronie's disease for sixteen months. Will the pain during ejaculation ever go away?

It is unusual for the pain associated with Peyronie's to last as long as sixteen months. It is possible that you have significant tethering of nerves in the scar tissue, which are stretched at the time of orgasm and ejaculation. If the pain is occurring only with ejaculation, it is also possible that there may be another cause for this pain, such as inflammation of the prostate. In this case, it would be best to seek an evaluation by a urologist who specializes in sexual dysfunction.

6. My erections seem shorter than normal, my penis seems more slender, and the head of my penis never gets firm. I assumed I had Peyronie's disease, but my doctor said there was no hard spot, which is typical of Peyronie's scarring. I am wondering if there could be another cause, such as low testosterone.

The scenario that you describe may be due to a diffuse scarring disorder involving the outer jacket of the penis rather than Peyronie's disease. With a diffuse scarring disorder, there is no palpable plaque, but the entire outer jacket or tunic has a loss of elasticity. Another possibility is that the scarring may involve the septum, which is the space or wall between the two erectile cylinders of the penis. Septal lesions are difficult to feel and these scars involving the center portion of the penis often cause shortening and may interfere with blood flow beyond the area of the scar, resulting in what is known as *distal flaccidity* or a softer shaft beyond the scar. Color dynamic duplex ultrasound evaluation of the penis may reveal scarring within the outer jacket of the penis and/or septum as well as within the penile vascular tissue.

The question as to whether testosterone may be a factor is also important as there is a common misconception that erectile dysfunction is due to low testosterone. In fact, low testosterone in the blood is rarely the cause of erectile insufficiency.

7. I have a slight curvature upward, a slight indentation in the middle of my shaft, and a small hard spot at the base. The hard spot and the pain started in the middle of the shaft, but have moved progressively to the base. Is this common?

This may be a very mild form of Peyronie's disease, and it is quite common for the plaque or nodular scar to seem as though it is moving. Basically this is part of the abnormal scarring process that occurs. The good news is that your deformity is "slight." You should be careful during sexual activity to avoid bending the penis excessively as this could activate the disease further.

8. My penis has a severe curvature towards the right when erect. It has an indentation at the base, as well. There is no pain when erect or flaccid. When I have sexual intercourse, only a part of my penis gets inserted. What can I do?

If the penis has always had a curvature, then it is unlikely that it is due to Peyronie's disease. It is more likely that this is a congenital abnormality. Congenital curvature of the penis is called chordee. If the curvature is so severe that it is interfering with penetrative sex, then you should see a urologist who is capable of surgically repairing this problem. If a new onset of deformity interferes with penetrative sex, then it would also be reasonable to see a urologist first since they are most likely to be familiar with Peyronie's disease and could offer the best advice. If complete insertion of the penis cannot be obtained, and it is not causing you or your partner any discomfort, then you can certainly make do with partial insertion.

3

Peyronie's Disease
and Sexual Function

Erectile dysfunction is associated with Peyronie's disease, but ED doesn't occur in all cases. In fact, some men with Peyronie's disease experience no problems engaging in sexual activity, including penetration. In some cases, however, the deformity can make it difficult to have sexual intercourse. In general, it depends on how severe your deformity is. For instance, if you have mild curvature, you may have no problem achieving an erection or engaging in penetrative sex. But if your curvature is severe, it may make it difficult to achieve an erection and to have sexual intercourse.

Likewise, minor indentations may not pose a problem, but severe indentations can lead to hinging or buckling of the penis, which can make sexual intercourse impossible. Shortening, although emotionally distressing, usually doesn't prevent you from having sexual intercourse.

1. If I have Peyronie's disease, should I avoid sexual intercourse altogether?

It depends. The most commonly recognized trigger activating Peyronie's disease is sexual activity. If pressures within the penis are higher than the penile tissues can withstand, it may cause excessive stretching and tearing, thereby activating the underlying abnormal wound-healing process. When Peyronie's disease is still in the acute stage (usually less than six to nine months) and there is pain when developing an erection, sexual activity should be minimized for comfort.

Once the pain felt with erections becomes tolerable or disappears, then sexual activity may resume. However, it's important to realize that another injury to the penis may occur, particularly if excessive forces are placed on the penis. This most commonly occurs when the female is on top or if there is rather vigorous intercourse with a mis-thrust causing sudden bending of the penis. Therefore, the best advice is to engage in careful intercourse so as to reduce the likelihood of an inadvertent re-injury.

2. Is it okay to masturbate if I have Peyronie's disease?

Masturbation certainly may allow sexual gratification, but if a strong erection occurs and the Peyronie's disease is still active, this may cause pain. It would be best to consider masturbation without trying to straighten the penis, which may cause increasing pressures and forces within the scar tissue and may cause more scarring to follow. Therefore, the bottom line is gentle and careful masturbation may be acceptable, but it's important to use common sense to avoid re-injuring the penis. Excessive forces may occur by pressing any object against the penis, which may cause bending or buckling, which could activate the Peyronie's scarring process.

3. My erections are softer since I developed Peyronie's disease. Should this happen? Is this normal?

Studies have shown that anywhere from 30 to 80 percent of men will report some reduction in the rigidity of their erections at the time of their initial examination by a doctor. Studies have also shown that the majority of men who have softening of their erections associated with Peyronie's disease will have this as a result of underlying vascular disease, which causes erectile dysfunction in men even without Peyronie's disease. Therefore, medical problems like diabetes, high blood pressure, elevated cholesterol, and smoking can all cause erectile dysfunction due to accelerated injury to the blood vessels within the penis. If you have Peyronie's disease and have one or more of these medical risk factors, it is more likely that you will have some erectile dysfunction as well.

It is also important to recognize that Peyronie's disease causes a good deal of emotional distress, and this distress may blunt or inhibit your sexual response. Therefore, a psychological form of erectile dysfunction occurs in up to 30 percent of men with diminished rigidity for understandable reasons. Lastly, there is some evidence that the deformity itself may cause changes in the penis that can result in diminished internal pressures, resulting in a softer erection.

Note: In my practice, up to 90 percent of the men I see with Peyronie's disease note some softening. Interestingly, 50 percent of the men I see in my practice develop their erectile dysfunction before developing Peyronie's disease and the other 50 percent after the Peyronie's disease occurred.

4. Along with the indentation and the lump in my penis in the flaccid state, I also have pain at times. I have trouble maintaining full erections. Do I risk causing further damage if I have sex?

It is unlikely that if you try to stimulate your penis without putting excessive stretching on the penis that you will worsen the Peyronie's disease. Sexual positions that might cause excessive stretching could reactivate or aggravate the acute inflammatory process, which would result in pain and possibly progressive deformity.

Peyronie's disease is manifest in the early phase with pain, which can be present in the flaccid state when touching the penis and more often when erect or trying to have intercourse. Typically, the pain will diminish with time. The pain and the deformity can result in psychological distress, which can interfere with your erection, but there may also be vascular changes, which may contribute to this as well.

5. Will Peyronie's disease interfere with my ability to impregnate my wife?

As a rule, Peyronie's disease doesn't interfere with your ability to impregnate a woman. However, if you are hoping to impregnate your partner, then it is best to have full penetration to deliver the seminal fluid and sperm into the depths of the vagina. If your deformity prevents you from achieving full insertion of your penis during intercourse, you may want to seek treatment.

6. As the result of a biking accident, I have erectile dysfunction and pain. Erections are rare without desire and my penis is curved upwards toward my body. I am 22. Do I suffer from PD?

The typical injury occurring with biking or any straddle sport is an injury to the vascular or nerve supply to the penis, which can result in erectile dysfunction and/or a numb penis. The fact that there is pain may indicate a nerve entrapment. If the deformity of the penis is new, there may also be scarring of the penile tissues resulting in the curvature. It appears that there may be both an erectile dysfunction problem here, which may be due to nerve and/or vessel injury, as well as a possible Peyronie's problem. Clearly, the best advice here is to see a local urologist for proper evaluation.

7. What kind of oral medications are available for erectile dysfunction if I also have Peyronie's disease?

Oral medications are typically the first course of action for treating men who have erectile dysfunction and PD. The most common oral medications are Viagra (*sildenafil citrate*), Levitra (*vardenafil*), and Cialis (*tadalafil*), none of which are likely to worsen Peyronie's disease.

Considering that up to 50 percent of men have ED prior to developing PD, many men are already taking these drugs.

8. What is MUSE and how does it treat erectile dysfunction if I also have Peyronie's disease?

MUSE (Medicated Urethral System for Erection) is a treatment for erectile dysfunction associated with Peyronie's disease, and may be recommended if oral medications fail. With MUSE, when you want to get an erection, you place a tiny pellet smaller than a grain of rice into the urethra using a thin tube as an applicator. The pellet contains a chemical known as *alprostadil*, which causes blood vessel dilation. When placed in the urethra, a small percentage of this drug will seep into the erectile tissue resulting in an erection. Alprostadil has been shown in experimental studies to potentially reduce scarring.

9. What is injection therapy for erectile dysfunction and can it cause Peyronie's disease?

Injection therapy for erectile dysfunction involves injecting medicine into the side of the shaft of the penis. The medications used in these injections may include alprostadil alone or in combination with other agents. One of the side effects associated with injection therapy is bruising. To reduce bruising, it is recommended that you keep the injection site compressed for three to five minutes following each injection. Another side effect when using injections is a potential increased risk of scarring. Most commonly, the scarring that occurs after penile injection therapy for ED is within the vascular erectile tissue and not in the outer jacket of the penis where Peyronie's develops. However, if the injection is placed directly into the Peyronie's plaque, it could pose more of a problem. Because of the increased risk for scarring, injection therapy is usually only recommended if other ED treatments have failed.

In spite of the increased risk for scarring, it is not likely that injection therapy used for the treatment of ED causes Peyronie's disease. However, because the injection therapy causes a stronger erection, you may be more apt to injure your penis during sexual intercourse. In the susceptible individual, this could activate the abnormal scarring process resulting in the Peyronie's deformity.

10. When I took Viagra, it gave me a full erection and made it possible for me to have sex. However, I have heard Viagra makes PD worse. Is this true?

The key point to remember is that if you have Peyronie's disease and you use Viagra or another oral erection drug to enhance your erections, it is possible that you could reinjure your penis during sex. It is therefore wise to be careful about your sexual activity in order to reduce the likelihood of recurrent trauma and reactivation of the Peyronie's process.

A published study examining the effects of Viagra in men with ED and PD demonstrated that it did improve erectile function in 71 percent of the men receiving Viagra. In addition, none of them had worsening of their deformity or new onset of pain. Furthermore, there is research evidence that Viagra, as well as the other oral erection drugs, can increase the amount of circulating nitric oxide, which appears in the research setting to have an anti-scarring effect.

Your question points out a misconception about the use of Viagra and the other *oral erection drugs*, such as Cialis and Levitra, often based on the package inserts that come with the drug. All three of the companies that manufacture oral erection drugs include a cautionary note in their package inserts, explaining that they did not specifically study ED in men with Peyronie's disease and therefore, they do not make any claims about its efficacy. This cautionary note is sometimes misinterpreted as meaning men with PD should not take the drugs.

11. Can oral erection drugs, such as Viagra, Levitra, or Cialis, improve my PD?

Using these medications may reduce the scarring process. That's because these drugs can increase the amount of nitric oxide within the penis. Nitric oxide is a chemical that is released by the penile nerves and blood vessels following sexual stimulation. This results in blood vessel dilation, increased blood flow, and erection. Studies have shown that an increase in nitric oxide within the penis may reduce the scarring associated with Peyronie's disease. It's doubtful that occasional use of these medications will result in any significant benefit with regard to the deformity, but several researchers and experts on Peyronie's disease are recommending the use of these drugs on a nightly or every-other-night basis due to their potential anti-scarring effect.

12. Does treatment of erectile dysfunction cause Peyronie's disease?

There are many misconceptions—even among physicians—that various treatments of erectile dysfunction cause Peyronie's disease. In fact, it is unlikely that any form of treatment for ED causes Peyronie's disease. At this time, there is no convincing evidence that the oral treatments for erectile dysfunction disease, such as Viagra, Levitra, or Cialis, cause Peyronie's disease. Similarly, there is no convincing evidence that the use of penile injection therapy or MUSE causes Peyronie's disease. It is more likely that these treatments provide a more rigid penis, which allows you to engage in sexual activity where the penis is at increased risk for injury.

13. Will the ED correct itself once I get treatment for the Peyronie's disease?

Occasionally, the erectile dysfunction may be due to the anxiety associated with the deformity. When treatment is initiated, the simple act of addressing the problem may be enough to relieve the anxiety that may have been affecting your sexual response. As a result, you may find the erections spontaneously getting better as you go through your treatment for Peyronie's disease.

14. Do penile enlargement pills and patches work?

Unfortunately, there is little evidence that any of the pills, potions, or patches advertised today provide any benefit whatsoever with regard to enhancement of penile girth or length. Nor are they expected to have any potential benefit in terms of treating penile deformities associated with Peyronie's disease. The Federal Government investigates companies for making false claims regarding sexual and penile enhancement.

Unfortunately, because the advertised agents are not submitted for FDA approval, the regulations to control them are not under the control of the FDA, but rather under the purview of the Federal Trade Commission (FTC). Therefore it may be up to the government to help control some of these companies that are taking advantage of many men who are in dire straits because of Peyronie's disease or who simply want to have a larger and longer penis. At this time, there is no reason to use any of these over-the-counter or Internet-advertised products. Their contents are largely unknown, and they could result in potential toxicity. In addition, they have not been shown to have any reliable benefit. The bottom line here is save your money.

15. I read that daily erections are crucial to bringing oxygen into the penile blood and tissues and to prevent collagen and subsequent scarring from forming. Is a lack of daily erections a problem? And if so, what can I do about it?

Daily erections are necessary for oxygenization of the penis, and a complete absence of erections can lead to erectile dysfunction. Penile oxygenization is the act of supplying oxygen to the penis. The penis goes from being in a low-oxygen state when flaccid to a high-oxygen state when erect, which shows that oxygenization is necessary in order to get an erection. In addition, oxygenization is crucial in order to maintain good vascular health within the penis. It is believed that this is why it is believed that men have nocturnal erectile activity. These erections occur due to a spontaneous reflex, which happens anywhere from two to seven times per night. This will in a sense "exercise" the penile vascular tissue by causing blood vessel dilation, better blood flow, and erection. This process nourishes the penile tissue and prevents collagen from forming. If collagen develops, it results in vascular tissue scarring with subsequent erectile dysfunction.

This is the scenario that is believed to occur following penile nerve injury at the time of radical prostate removal for prostate cancer. In an effort to rehabilitate the penis following this surgery and to prevent erectile dysfunction, men are encouraged to take oral medication such as Viagra, Levitra, or Cialis at night to encourage nocturnal erections and/or to use drugs which are instilled into the urethra or injected directly into the penis to stimulate erection.

Part II

Nonsurgical Treatment

4

Oral Medications

Peyronie's disease may affect your sex life, your self-esteem, and your mood. It's understandable that you may feel desperate to find a remedy. Over the years, hundreds of therapies have been tried, but there is still no known cure for this condition. Even so, there are a number of nonsurgical treatment options currently available that may provide some welcome relief and improvement.

Nonsurgical treatment, often in the form or medications, is often the first course of action prescribed, and in many cases it can reduce symptoms and lead to better sexual function. You may find that taking action to fight the disease can also improve your mood and relieve some of the anxiety you may be feeling. Even if nonsurgical remedies don't provide you with ideal results, they won't prevent you from being able to take advantage of more advanced therapies, such as surgery, at a later date.

1. What oral therapies currently available show the most promise for treating Peyronie's disease?

Pentoxifylline is a prescription drug that has been used to increase blood flow, particularly in the lower extremities in patients who have vascular disease. It has also been suggested that it may reduce the formation of scar tissue and therefore may have some beneficial effect in patients with Peyronie's disease. It is an inexpensive generic drug, but it is inconvenient since it should be taken three times per day.

L-arginine is an amino acid and a precursor to nitric oxide. It appears that in situations of chronic scarring, elevated levels of nitric oxide may have a beneficial anti-scarring effect. L-arginine is the most promising over-the-counter remedy currently available.

Phosphodiesterase type 5 (PDE5) inhibitors (Viagra, Levitra, and Cialis) have been shown in the research laboratory to reduce the growth rate of the cells that make scar tissue. In research studies on Peyronie's disease using animals, these medications were given to animals in their drinking water. The animals were then injected with a drug to cause a Peyronie's disease-like scar. The animals that received any of these three medications had a reduced amount of scar tissue as compared to the animals that did not receive these medications. Therefore, theoretically these agents can be used on a nightly or every-other-nightly basis not only to improve erectile function, but also to possibly reduce scarring. These are prescription drugs and must be used with caution as there are potential side effects.

2. What oral therapies do you recommend?

Current oral medication regimens being recommended may include pentoxifylline three times daily, L-arginine 500 mg two times daily, and for those men who may have some erectile insufficiency and can afford these expensive medications, nightly or every-other-nightly Viagra 50 mg, Levitra 10 mg, or Cialis 10 mg. Again, these treatments should be administered by a physician to ensure that you do not have any reason not to take them.

3. Can taking calcium pills for any length of time cause calcification of the plaque?

There is no evidence that taking calcium as a supplement would encourage calcification of a Peyronie's plaque. Any calcification of the plaque likely occurs due to genetics. It is unlikely that the calcification process is altered by taking extra calcium or by avoiding taking calcium.

4.   Are there any oral treatments that aren't recommended?

Vitamin E is the most frequently used drug by both primary care physicians and urologists for treatment of Peyronie's disease. Use of Vitamin E is based upon studies performed in the 1950s, which suggested some improvement of scarring and deformity. Unfortunately, no study since that time has demonstrated any real benefit and the best clinical trial performed in 1983 demonstrated no benefit at all. Therefore, although Vitamin E may have some beneficial effects as an antioxidant and may potentially reduce the risk of lung, colon, and prostate cancer, it is not recommended for Peyronie's disease. Despite this, many doctors still recommend the use of Vitamin E at anywhere from 400 to 2,000 mg daily. However, using doses higher than 400 mg daily carries the risk of toxicity. If you choose to take Vitamin E, use no more than 400 mg daily.

Potaba, or potassium amino-benzoate, has been around for many years. It is a prescription drug used for Peyronie's disease as well as for other ailments. It is unclear as to how Potaba works and recently a reputable *placebo-controlled trial* in Europe demonstrated reduction in plaque size but no meaningful change in penile deformity. (A placebo is an inert substance used in controlled experiments to test the efficacy of another drug. In a controlled study, one group receives the real drug; the other group receives the placebo. This assists in understanding whether the treatment is truly providing some benefit.) Unfortunately, there are a good deal of gastrointestinal side effects, and it is an expensive drug, requiring up to twenty-four tablets to be taken daily. Therefore, Potaba is not recommended.

Colchicine was introduced in the 1990s as a potential anti-fibrotic agent that might interfere with the scarring process. Animal studies suggested some benefit, but placebo-controlled trials have not shown any benefit. It is a generic drug and therefore inexpensive, but it does cause significant gastrointestinal side effects and, in the rare individual, might even shut down the bone marrow for production of red and white blood cells.

Tamoxifen is an oral anti-estrogen agent, the same agent used in treating breast cancer, that has been shown to be beneficial in treating a form of scar formation that occurs in the tissues that reside behind the bowels. Placebo-controlled trials performed in Brazil showed no benefit and several of the men had hair loss, known as *alopecia*. Therefore, tamoxifen is not recommended.

Carnitine is an oral agent that has been suggested to be beneficial to men with Peyronie's disease, but it is unclear exactly how or why. No placebo-controlled trials have been performed, but carnitine has been compared to tamoxifen.

Allegra (*fexofenadine*) is an antihistamine. To date, no formal studies have been performed to examine the use of this agent for the treatment of any Peyronie's disease symptom whatsoever. It is possible that anecdotal reports are circulating by either physicians or individuals who are trying these products randomly, but there is no known rationale as to why these agents would work, and no studies to support their use.

Oral Medications Used for Peyronie's Disease

Name	How It Works	Side Effects	Efficacy
Vitamin E	Antioxidant	Very few except at doses greater than 400 mg	None shown in placebo-controlled trials
Potaba	Unclear	Gastrointestinal distress, nausea, must take up to twenty-four tablets daily	None shown for reducing penile deformity in placebo-controlled trial; may make plaque smaller
Colchicine	May inhibit growth rate of scar-making cells	Gastrointestinal distress, possible bone marrow suppression	None shown in placebo-controlled trial
Tamoxifen	Anti-fibrotic and anti-estrogen	Gastrointestinal distress, hair loss	None shown in placebo-controlled trial
Carnitine	Unknown, may increase oxygen content in tissue	None	None shown
Pentoxifylline	May reduce scar by blocking proteins that cause scarring	Few noted, nausea, dizziness	Only one case report currently available but makes scientific sense
L-arginine	Precursor to nitric oxide which acts as an anti-scarring agent	None	No trials showing benefit

5

Topical Treatments

Any treatment that is applied to the skin overlying the Peyronie's plaque is defined as a topical therapy. This includes various drugs, chemicals, and procedures that may be applied directly to the skin in the hope that they will penetrate into the underlying scar tissue and diminish pain, plaque size, and deformity.

Topical treatments include gels, iontophoresis, which is electrical stimulation, shock waves, and others.

1. How are topical gels used to treat PD?

Topical gels are drugs that are applied to the surface of the penile skin over the plaque. Many have been used historically, but currently the most popular one is topical *verapamil* gel. Verapamil is a calcium channel blocker. Calcium channel blockers are known to change the way certain cells behave. For example, if cells within scar tissue are exposed to an adequate concentration of verapamil (much more than can be achieved by oral administration), the cells may stop making scar tissue, and in fact may break down scar tissue instead.

There are multiple formulations of topical verapamil, but only one has been patented. None of the formulations have been approved by the FDA because none of them have undergone proper clinical trials, however, they can still be used for treatment. The gel is combined with a skin-penetrating agent that is designed to carry the verapamil through the skin to the underlying scar tissue. Unfortunately, it has not yet been shown whether the verapamil makes it to the underlying plaque in adequate concentrations to result in a beneficial change. Therefore, topical verapamil gels cannot be recommended at this time as there really isn't evidence to show penetration to underlying tissues, nor are there any reports showing measured improvement.

2.   What is iontophoresis (EMDA)?

Iontophoresis, also known as Electromotive Drug Administration (EMDA), is a noninvasive, painless therapy in which an electric current is delivered to the penile skin overlying the plaque. The electric current is designed to carry drugs, such as verapamil and dexamethasone, into the underlying scar tissue in an effort to reduce its size. *Dexamethasone* is a steroid that is an anti-inflammatory and anti-scarring agent. Several clinical trials have shown that iontophoresis may potentially reduce the scar tissue in patients with Peyronie's disease. Most of the clinical studies performed on iontophoresis have shown some benefit when verapamil and dexamethasone are used together anywhere from two to four times per week

A published study in men who received verapamil by EMDA prior to having their plaques excised surgically, demonstrated that up to 70 percent of those individuals had measurable verapamil in their plaques. Therefore, it appears that EMDA can deliver the drugs to the underlying tissue. The question remains: is the level high enough to bring about the desired change in the scar tissue? Another EMDA study of verapamil versus saline found that both groups showed some benefit in curvature. This suggested that perhaps the electric current itself had some beneficial properties and resulted in some wound healing.

3.   What kind of results can be achieved with iontopheresis?

Overall, the results from EMDA show an average of 10-15 degrees of improvement in penile curvature in those men who respond. There also appears to be a rapid resolution of pain and some reduction in plaque size. Because of this, EMDA is recommended for use in patients who have mild curvature (less than 45 degrees) and who have an active plaque with painful erections.

Note: My experience with this device is that 50 to 60 percent of treated men have mild improvement of their erectile deformity ranging from 5 to 30 degrees, with an average improvement of about 10 degrees. Therefore, this approach typically isn't used in men who have more advanced curvature, unless they are also experiencing a good deal of pain. This treatment option has been shown to accelerate resolution of pain.

4. How is iontophoresis administered? Do I have to go to my doctor's office for it or can I do it at home?

Iontophoresis can be administered in a doctor's office, but you'll likely be advised to purchase a device so you can do it yourself in the privacy of your own home. Your doctor can provide you with information on where to purchase a device and how to use it. In general, two to four treatments per week are recommended, with each treatment taking twenty minutes. Be aware that the devices are costly, with a full setup including drugs costing about $1,200. The devices most commonly recommended by doctors are manufactured by Physion in Italy.

5. I found numerous companies that make portable devices similar to Physion's device. Are all these machines basically the same?

At this time it does not appear that all iontophoresis devices are the same.

The Physion device is unique. It delivers the positively charged energy via a reservoir cup, which is filled with the verapamil with or without the dexamethasone solution and attached with an adhesive

Electromotive Drug Administration (EMDA)

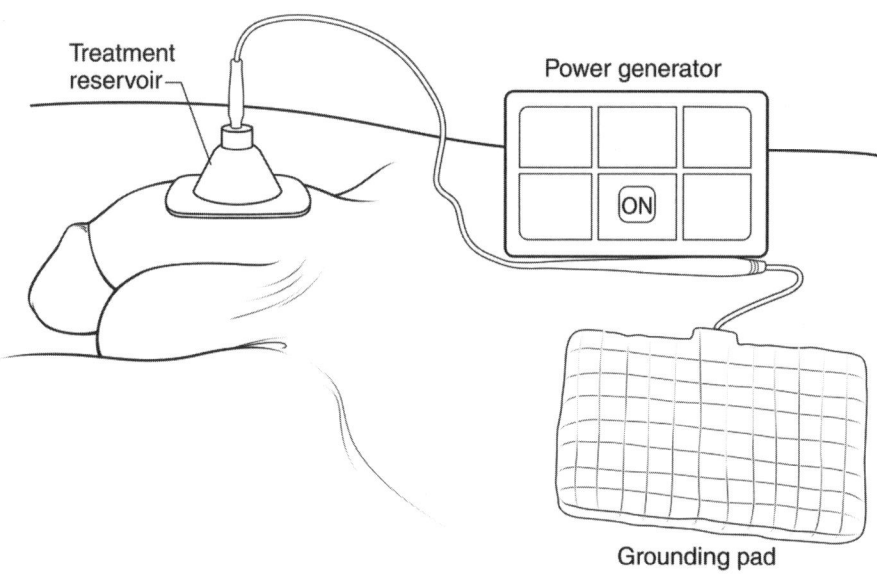

The apparatus for electromotive drug administration (EMDA), also known as iontophoresis, is shown here. It delivers drugs, intended to reduce scar tissue, through a low-level electrical current.

agent over the scar on the penis. On the other hand, the other iontophoresis devices on the market use a pad that is saturated with the drug being administered, such as verapamil. Presently, no studies have been done on patients with Peyronie's disease that demonstrate that these other devices result in actual transfer of the drug into the underlying plaque. One study did show that with the Physion device, 71 percent of patients had measurable levels of verapamil within their plaque when this procedure was performed.

6. Is there anyone who shouldn't use iontophoresis?

Iontophoresis may not be recommended for patients with downward curvature. If you have downward curvature, your plaque is located on the underside of the penis, which is also where the urethra is located. Because of this, it is difficult to get exposure to the underlying plaque through the urethra.

7. What is shock-wave therapy?

Shock waves have been used since the 1980s as a form of treatment for kidney and gallbladder stones. This is a noninvasive therapy that directs a shock wave, typically generated by a spark plug, to pass through the skin and focus on a target. If you have Peyronie's disease, the target is the plaque within the penis. Special shock-wave machines have been developed to treat scars and calcifications, particularly in the shoulder and in the foot. They have been successful in reducing pain and improving function of the shoulder and foot. As a result, some urologists, primarily in Europe, have used shock-waves as a treatment for Peyronie's disease.

Unfortunately, in the multiple studies that have been published, the acceptable criteria for success have not been met. More recent studies have not shown any benefit to shock-wave therapy. It has also been suggested that shockwaves may cause more scarring, particularly on the opposite side of the penis which might cause a false straightening, and may also cause further shortening of the penis. At this point, shock-wave therapy cannot be recommended, and most of the European countries are no longer paying for shock-wave therapy for Peyronie's disease in their national health programs.

8. What about other topical treatments such as energy therapy?

Energy therapy is a form of treatment that employs various forms of energy, such as ultrasound or lasers, to try to drive a drug into the scar tissue to help minimize it, or possibly uses the energy alone to activate the healing process within the established scar. Unfortunately, studies have not demonstrated any benefit with either of these treatments alone or in combination with any drug to reduce the deformity of a Peyronie's plaque.

9.   Is acupuncture effective in treating Peyronie's disease?

At this point, there have been no studies performed using acupuncture for the treatment of Peyronie's disease. It is certainly possible that acupuncture may reduce the pain associated with Peyronie's disease as it has been found to be a successful treatment for a variety of pain syndromes. With regard to any improvement of penile deformity, it's unclear how acupuncture could help, but stranger things have been reported. At this time, acupuncture is not recommended for the improvement of penile deformity associated with Peyronie's disease.

10.   Will topical or oral chelation agents have any affect on PD, as it dissolves plaque in the arteries?

There are no formal studies that have been done on liquid or oral *chelation* products. Chelation is the act of drawing properties, such as calcium, out of the body through urination or defecation. Although patients have suggested that there has been some improvement or reduction of calcification of plaque as a result of using chelation agents, this is totally unproven and, frankly, not likely. There would be no reason whatsoever to use any chelation agent when the plaque is not calcified.

6

Injection Therapy

Injection therapy, also known as *intralesional injection therapy*, means that a drug is being injected directly into the lesion or scar tissue. The intent is to stop the production of scar tissue. How do these agents do this? All cells in the body rely on calcium to function. If you block the calcium channels, calcium cannot flow in and out of the cell, which can cause changes in cell function. In the case of Peyronie's disease, the goal is to change the behavior of the cells responsible for making scar tissue.

1. How do injections work to treat PD?

For injection therapy, verapamil is the drug used. This drug is primarily known as a calcium channel blocker. High concentrations of verapamil may cause the cells to stop making scar tissue and cause them to start breaking down scar tissue instead. This has yet to be proven in the laboratory in patients with Peyronie's disease.

As of the current time, verapamil seems to be the most sensible and scientifically sound drug to use as treatment for Peyronie's disease as a topical or injectable agent. However, it should not be considered a cure as it will not result in complete resolution of the scar or deformity. But, since it can result in some improvement when administered properly, it may be a treatment option you should discuss with your doctor.

Note: In 1992, I was the first doctor to introduce verapamil as a treatment for Peyronie's disease. Since that time, more than 800 men have been treated and about 40 to 60 percent have measured improvement of curvature ranging from 10 to 75 degrees.

2. How are injections given? Are they painful?

Injection therapy should not hurt if the penis is properly anesthetized prior to the injection of the drug. The initial injection of a numbing medicine, known as Marcaine, may cause a temporary burning sensation, but this tends to dissipate quickly. It may take anywhere from ten to twenty minutes for the penis to become completely numb, at which point the injectable drug can be administered with almost no discomfort at all. Occasionally, there will be a sense of pressure. If there is still pain, a second injection of the anesthetic can be given. The anesthetic is administered with a small-gauge needle around the base of the penis where the nerves emerge out of the deep pelvis.

3. How often are verapamil intralesional injections given and how quickly should I see a response?

Typically, an injection is given every two weeks for up to twelve injections. The changes that occur with intralesional injection or any nonsurgical therapy of Peyronie's disease may not take place rapidly. This is because once scar tissue is established, it is difficult to initiate a remodeling process. And if scar remodeling is going to occur at all, it is unlikely to occur quickly. However, some men have noticed an improvement in their deformity after receiving their first injection of verapamil. This is typically a small improvement.

The hope is that over the course of a series of injections, incremental improvement will occur. In some cases, progressive improvement is noted over the course of several injections and then stabilization without improvement is noted over the course of several subsequent injections. This is not an unusual scenario. The goal of injection therapy with verapamil is that improvement will be noted at the end of the series of twelve injections and that improvement will continue even after the injection therapy sessions stop. However, if after six injections there is no improvement whatsoever, it is recommended that this treatment be stopped.

4. What if I don't see any improvement from the injection therapy with verapamil? Should I undergo a second series of injections?

Unfortunately, when a man goes through injection therapy with verapamil and there is no visible improvement in the deformity of the erect penis following a course of six injections, then further injection is unlikely to result in any substantial benefit. In some instances, a higher dose of verapamil may be recommended as a way to enhance the results. If a higher dosage of verapamil still doesn't produce beneficial results, then additional injection therapy isn't advised.

5. While undergoing intralesional verapamil injections, my plaque appears to have gotten bigger. Is this normal and should I stop treatment?

In most patients, the plaque becomes slightly larger during the course of intralesional injections of verapamil. It is unclear why this occurs, but it may be because of local inflammation as well as the volume of fluid that is injected into the scar tissue. The plaque may appear to become thicker or larger during the course of treatment, but once injection therapy stops, the plaque will get progressively smaller. This typically occurs over the first six months following the end of injection therapy.

In addition, the greatest concern here is not so much what the plaque is doing but whether the penile deformity in the erect state is improving. Even though the plaque may appear to be larger, the penis in the erect state may show improvement. If, after six injections, the plaque is bigger and there is no improvement whatsoever in the

Drug Injection Therapy

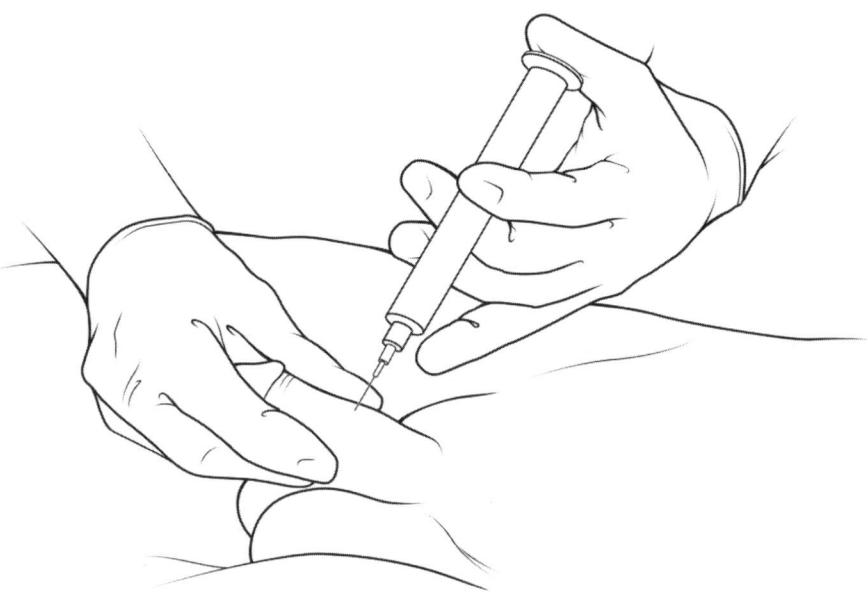

Intralesional drug injections, given to reduce curvature, are delivered directly into the plaque after the penis is numbed with a long-acting anesthetic.

deformity—such as reduced curvature, increased girth, resolution of pain, or improved quality of erections—then injection therapy with verapamil should be stopped.

6. If I see some improvement as a result of injection therapy with verapamil, what are the chances that I will have a recurrence of Peyronie's disease symptoms at a later time?

In the past decade or so, many papers on verapamil injections have been published in medical journals stating that no recurrences have been reported in men who have experienced improvement or even stabilization of their Peyronie's disease. It is certainly possible that a man who has undergone injection therapy could have a recurrence as a result of a reinjury, but again this has not been reported. It is unclear why Peyronie's disease has not recurred following treatment with verapamil. It could be due to a change in the behavior of the penile tissue, such that it is less likely to be traumatized. It could be that Peyronie's disease is a "one-shot deal" that, once stabilized, is unlikely to recur. Or, it could be that men who have Peyronie's disease are more apt to be careful during sexual activity, which would reduce their likelihood of injury during sex.

7. What is interferon, and when is it used for injection therapy?

Sometimes used in injection therapy, *interferon* is a drug made up of naturally occurring proteins that are produced by the immune system. Interferon helps the body's immune system attack viruses, bacteria, and tumors. This action slows or blocks the attacking "invader" cells.

Interferon has been shown to have similar properties to verapamil in terms of changing the behavior of the scar-making tissues in the Peyronie's plaque. Multiple studies have been conducted over the past decade, but most did not show any substantial benefit. One study, however, did demonstrate some improvement in deformity, pain, and plaque size when using interferon. On the downside, interferon is far more expensive than verapamil and has been associated with side effects similar to what you might experience with the flu, including muscle aches, fever, and general malaise or feeling badly. These symptoms are typically mild to moderate and may be relieved by taking an anti-inflammatory drug, such as ibuprofen.

8. How often are interferon intralesional injections given and how quickly should I see a response?

Typically, an injection is given every two weeks for up to twelve injections. The hope is that over the course of a series of injections, incremental improvement will occur. In some cases, progressive improvement is noted over the course of several injections and then stabilization without improvement is noted over the course of several subsequent injections. This is not an unusual scenario. The goal of injection therapy with interferon is that improvement will be noted at the end of the series of twelve injections and that improvement will continue even after the injection therapy sessions stop. However, if after six injections there is no improvement whatsoever, it is recommended that this treatment be stopped. These injections typically cost $250 to $300 per injection.

9. If I have some improvement from injection therapy with interferon, what are the chances that I will have a recurrence of Peyronie's disease at a later time?

The only study conducted on interferon that actually showed improvement of curvature had a short-term follow-up period, and it didn't include any data about recurrence. For this reason, it's difficult to determine the likelihood of experiencing a second episode of Peyronie's disease following injection therapy with interferon.

10. I have had Peyronie's disease for almost two years and just went through interferon injections every two weeks for three months. I have not seen any change. The Peyronie's specialist wants to do a second course of injections. If this did not work at all, do you think it is wise to go through a second battery of injections?

If you see no improvement in the deformity of the erect penis following a course of six injections with interferon, then you are unlikely to see any substantial benefit from further injections. Men receiving injection therapy with verapamil may be encouraged to try a higher dosage of verapamil in an effort to enhance improvements, but it is unclear at this time whether higher doses of interferon will produce any benefit. Most likely, your doctor will recommend a different type of treatment.

11. What are the side effects of injection therapy?

The potential side effects may include pain if the anesthesia is not sufficient, but this tends to be temporary at worst. In addition, there could be bruising on the skin, which occurs as a result of puncturing the blood vessels under the penile skin. This tends to resolve quickly, within a week to ten days, and leaves no long-term side effect. In a very small number of patients, verapamil injections will produce prolonged aching of the penis after the injection or some temporary numbness.

Note: In virtually all the patients I have treated since 1992, these side effects resolve. In patients receiving verapamil, there is the possible side effect of low blood pressure or a slower heart rate, but this has not been seen in more than 800 patients treated. For interferon, flu-like symptoms including muscle aches and pains, low-grade fever, and a general bad feeling has been reported.

12. Can men who are on aspirin, Coumadin, or Plavix undergo injection therapy?

Virtually all of the treatments currently available for Peyronie's disease can be offered to patients who are taking blood thinners, including Coumadin. The primary concern in using injection therapy is bruising, which may be worsened by the use of blood thinners. To reduce bruising, compression of the injection site should be maintained for at least ten minutes following the injection.

13. What is collagenase and is it being used for injection therapy?

Collagenase is an enzyme that is responsible for breaking down scar tissue during the normal wound-healing process. Wound healing occurs in three phases: the "cleanup" phase in which the damaged or dead tissue is removed, the active "scar formation" phase in which a heaped-up scar pulls the damaged tissues together, and the "scar remodeling" phase which is activated by collagenase and other enzymes to reorganize the big scar down to a thin, barely identifiable scar. Unfortunately, this normal wound-healing process doesn't occur if you have Peyronie's disease, and a lack of collagenase may be part of the reason why. Collagenase breaks down collagen, which is the primary component of a Peyronie's plaque.

In the 1980s, small scale studies were performed to determine whether collagenase injections into PD plaques would reduce curvature; however, the studies were not submitted to the FDA. Still, some men had substantial improvement in their curvatures and few had any

Injectable Drugs Used for Peyronie's Disease

Name	How It Works	Side Effects	Efficacy
Steroids (ie; Dexamethasone, Kenalog)	Anti-fibrotic, anti-inflammatory	Tissue atrophy (thinning) and disruption of normal surgical tissue planes, bruising	None shown in controlled trials
Verapamil	Reduces multiplication and growth of scar-making cells (fibroblasts), reduces collagen production	Potential reduced blood pressure yet no published evidence in patients with Peyronie's, bruising	40-60 % have reduction in curvature with average improvement around 25 degrees
Interferon alpha-2b	Biological modifier similar to verapamil	Flu-like symptoms, malaise, local pain, bruising	27% of men in one trial showed 12-degree reduction in curvature

serious side effects. Studies are ongoing to determine whether it may be useful to inject collagenase into PD plaques.

14. Can steroids be used in injection therapy?

Injection therapy began in the 1950s with the injection of steroids into the plaque. The use of cortisone, or any form of steroid injections for Peyronie's disease, was most commonly used in the 1960s through the early 1980s. Theoretically, steroids will reduce scar formation by inhibiting *fibroblasts* (scar-making cells) from making collagen, one of the primary components of scar tissue. But they can also cause thinning of the tissue, known as tissue *atrophy*, which weakens the tissues and can result in the disappearance of the space that is normally found between the nerves and the blood vessels that lie over the plaque.

If the steroid injection therapy treatment fails, which it does often, this may make other treatment options, such as surgery, more difficult to perform and less likely to produce a satisfactory result. In fact, it can put the penile tissues at increased risk for diminished blood flow and can lead to penile numbness if nerves are damaged. Therefore, steroids are not recommended for use with injection therapy. And although there are physicians, who may still be using steroid injection, it is not advisable since better and safer alternatives, such as verapamil and interferon, are currently available. In some instances, steroids may be used in combination with verapamil during topical therapy EMDA for selected patients.

15. Have there been any studies on using steroids in injection therapy?

The primary concern with steroid injection, as with many of the treatments for Peyronie's disease, is that virtually all of the studies in the past were flawed. For example, they were performed with a limited number of patients whose improvement was only reported subjectively without any measurements documenting reduction of deformity. In addition, the studies were not controlled with a placebo group. When there is no placebo group, the efficacy of the real drug cannot be proven.

16. Can Botox work at relaxing and softening Peyronie's plaque?

Botox is a agent that is currently used to reduce facial wrinkles by temporarily paralyzing underlying facial muscle tissues directly beneath the wrinkles. There is no evidence that Botox has a beneficial effect on Peyronie's disease.

7

Stretching Therapy

Stretching therapy is a type of treatment that is used in an effort to reduce the penile deformity associated with Peyronie's disease. The concept of penile stretching is similar to the concept of straightening your teeth with braces. It would seem that stretching the penis might result in a remodeling of tissue or change in the configuration of the Peyronie's scar. The problem is being able to provide prolonged pressure to the penis so that such a change could occur. To provide prolonged traction, two types of stretching devices are used to treat Peyronie's disease: an external vacuum device and an external penile extender device.

1. What is vacuum therapy, and how does it work?

Vacuum therapy is a type of stretching therapy that uses suction in an effort to reduce penile curvature. Vacuum therapy is applied with a specially designed vacuum cylinder into which the penis is placed. The vacuum is created by activating a pumping mechanism. The suction creates an erection, which stretches the Peyronie's plaque. The erect penis fills the vacuum tube and presses against the inner wall of the cylinder. The cylinder wall resists the curvature of the penis, thus creating a straightening, stretching force on the penis.

2. How often should I use a vacuum therapy device? Is it recommended that I use it with other treatments?

It is recommended that vacuum devices be used once or twice a day in a progressive fashion until you can tolerate leaving the device in place for thirty minutes. It is best to increase the intensity level of the vacuum gradually as you become accustomed to it. Gradual, sustained stretching for up to thirty minutes is ideal. Using a high-intensity pulse of vacuum in short bursts, say for only five minutes, is not useful. In fact, the abrupt nature of short bursts of high intensity may not be beneficial and may potentially cause injury. For your safety, the device can only be left on for thirty minutes at a time. Beyond that time, a low blood-flow state may occur, which could damage the vascular tissue of the penis.

It is usually recommended that vacuum therapy be used together with other medical treatments, such as injection therapy with verapamil. Verapamil is a drug that may cause cells to stop making scar tissue and cause them to start breaking down scar tissue instead. Vacuum therapy is currently being used together with verapamil injection therapy as a treatment option in an effort to combine the beneficial chemical effects of the verapamil with the mechanical stretching forces of the vacuum. As to whether long-term treatment with vacuum therapy alone or in combination with other medical therapy will benefit patients is yet to be proven.

3. Is there any proof that vacuum therapy works?

As of yet there is no documented evidence that vacuum therapy provides any benefit. Although it may appear to straighten the penis while the vacuum is in use, this straightening may not be long-lasting. It appears that the straightening experienced with the vacuum on is due to the expansion of tissues covering the plaque. As a result, a masking effect of the deformity occurs, producing what appears to be a more full and straight penis.

Vacuum therapy has been considered a potentially beneficial treatment for Peyronie's disease for many years. Some believe that stretching the penile tissue on a regular basis encourages a reduction in scar tissue, thus straightening the penis. And many physicians and patients have reported that they have seen improvements with regular use of a vacuum device. Concrete answers about whether or not vacuum therapy can actually help straighten the penis should be forthcoming after the completion of studies to test vacuum therapy.

4. Can vacuum therapy also be used to correct erectile dysfunction?

External vacuum devices have also been used as a treatment for erectile dysfunction. In fact, these devices have been used for more than one-hundred years to create an erect-like state. Penile vacuum therapy draws blood into the penis to create an erection, but it is not a true erection because as soon as the device is removed or the vacuum is released, the penis goes back to its flaccid state. To maintain the erection, a constriction band is placed around the base of the penis, at which point the vacuum device can be removed and the penis can be used for sexual intercourse. One potential concern is that if the constriction band is placed directly over the plaque, it may cause pain and may make it difficult to get a good seal, resulting in an inadequate erection.

5. Are there other possible side effects of using the vacuum device for penile straightening?

A common side effect of using a vacuum device is the appearance of tiny black-and-blue areas, which are an indication of the rupture of small blood vessels within the skin of the penis. These are typically painless and should go away within several days. In some cases, you may notice a collection of fluid under the skin. This is called *edema.* This fluid accumulation occurs as a result of the vacuum and again,

Vaccum Therapy

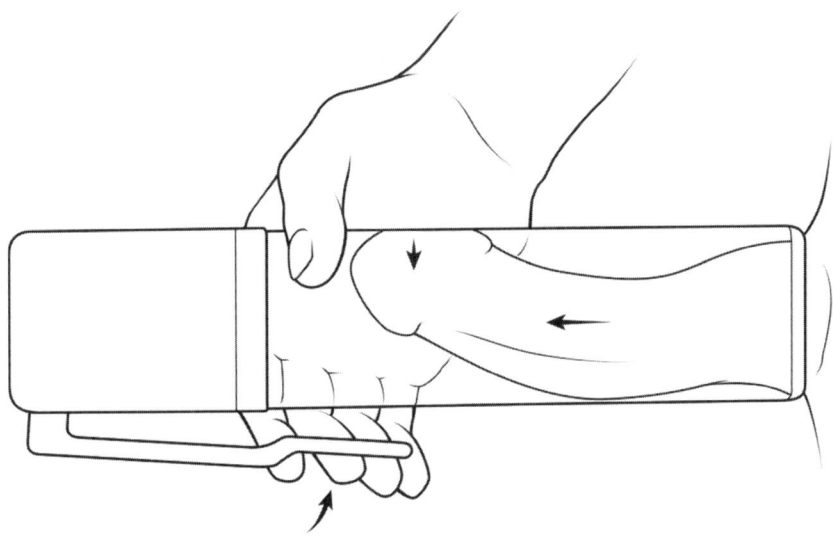

Vacuum therapy is used to straighten the penis and stretch scar tissue in an effort to reduce curvature. There is no scientific evidence that vacuum therapy works; however, many men and physicians believe regular stretching produces improvement.

tends to go away within twenty-four hours once the vacuum is released. This fluid accumulation poses no danger so long as it goes away on its own and so long as there is no evidence of any damage to the skin.

If you experience significant pain while using the vacuum, then the pressure should be reduced to a more tolerable level. You can build up your ability to tolerate the pressure over an extended period of time. Again, remember that the vacuum should not remain on the penis for longer than thirty minutes.

6. How do I obtain a vacuum device?

Vacuum devices are available with a prescription from your doctor or can be purchased over the counter. Before using a vacuum device, you should be evaluated by a physician who has experience treating Peyronie's disease. Based on this evaluation, your doctor would be able to prescribe the proper device. These prescription devices cost anywhere from $250 to $500. Over-the-counter devices are cheaper, but since they aren't controlled or regulated in terms of the amount of pressure that is obtained, it is advisable to pay more for a prescription device.

7. Can vacuum therapy hurt my penis or make my PD worse?

There are a few cases in the medical literature indicating that Peyronie's disease was activated when vacuum therapy was used. It is more likely that this occurred during sexual activity following the use of vacuum therapy to achieve an erection. An erection achieved using vacuum therapy can be maintained by placing a special constricting band on the penis after the vacuum tube is removed. It is likely that the vacuum itself did not cause the Peyronie's disease, but by providing a stronger erection, an injury was triggered during sexual activity, and activated the underlying disease in the susceptible individual. For the most part, if the vacuum device is used as directed, is applied carefully with a gradual increase of pressure over time, and is not used for longer than thirty minutes at a time, the likelihood of activating or worsening your Peyronie's disease is extremely low.

Note: In my experience with about fifty men using vacuum tubes for the correction of deformity associated with Peyronie's disease, no man has had worsening of their curvature as a result of this form of treatment, and many felt that the vacuum helped straighten their penis.

8. Can men who are on aspirin, Coumadin, or Plavix undergo vacuum therapy?

Yes, it is okay to undergo vacuum therapy if you are taking blood thinners. However, if you are considering the use of vacuum therapy in combination with injection therapy using verapamil and/or interferon, there are certain guidelines you should follow. For example, you must be very careful not to initiate vacuum therapy for at least forty-eight hours after an injection of verapamil and/or interferon. This is to prevent the pressure of the vacuum therapy from causing any significant subcutaneous bleeding. Should bruising occur following use of the vacuum, manual pressure can be applied directly over the black-and-blue area. With subsequent use of the vacuum device, a lower vacuum pressure should be used.

9. What is a penile extender or traction device?

Penile extenders are external devices that are designed to stretch the penis in hopes of straightening the penis. Unlike vacuum therapy devices that use suction to create an erection, penile extenders simply stretch the penis. A commonly used stretching device is the FastSize penile extender system. This is an external stretching device that is applied to the penis and must be worn for two to eight hours per day for up to six months. (The device should be removed for a few minutes every two hours; then it can be reattached.) The prolonged stretching forces are applied to the penis in an effort to cause remodeling and stretching of the scar tissue in hopes of straightening the penis.

10. Do penis extenders help with Peyronie's disease?

The use of a penile extender or stretching device has a similar goal to that of a vacuum device, which is to try to apply stretching forces to the penis to encourage remodeling of the scar tissue and straightening of the curved penis. It seems intuitive that if you can straighten teeth by applying continual forces with braces, than you might get this same type

Penile Extender
(Stretching Device)

of benefit from applying prolonged stretching forces to the curved penis. The problem is how much force can be applied, how to apply it, and how to apply it without causing injury.

Preliminary reports from patients in one study indicate positive changes in curvature, length, girth, and sexual function. Objective measures have revealed reduced curvature of 10 to 30 degrees and length gain of one-fourth to three-fourths of an inch. Until the complete results of this study are known, it is advisable to use an external penile stretching device only when recommended by a qualified physician after a full consultation and examination.

Note: I am currently recommending this stretching device together with pentoxifylline and L-arginine orally as well as intralesional verapamil injections every two weeks for six months as the most aggressive nonsurgical treatment of PD.

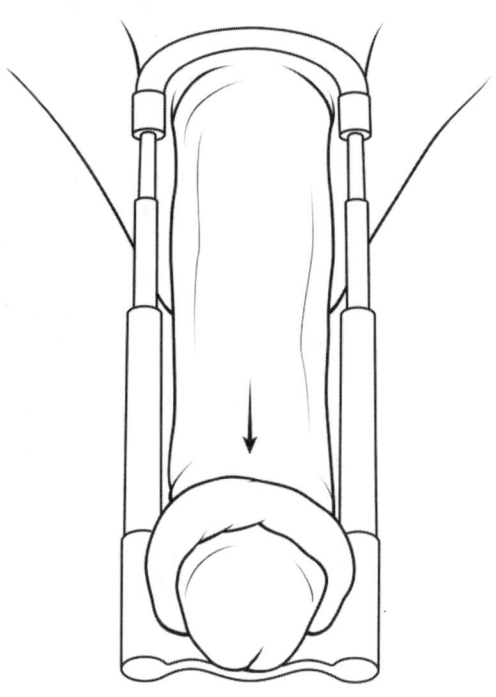

Similar to the vacuum, the penile extender is used to stretch scar tissue in the penis, causing remodeling and elongation. The device must be worn two to eight hours a day for six months. Some physicians report the device can reduce curvature.

8

Combination Therapy

When you use more than a single method of treatment for Peyronie's disease, it's called combination therapy. For example, you may consider receiving intralesional injections of verapamil along with an external stretching device or vacuum device at home on days when an injection is not given. Other combinations for Peyronie's disease can include oral therapy with injection therapy and iontophoresis (EMDA) with injection therapy and/or an external stretching device. Although these approaches may take six months or more before any benefit is seen, it's understandable that you might prefer combination therapy to surgery as a treatment option.

1. What combination of treatments are commonly recommended for PD?

If you have mild deformity, say 30 degrees or less, but still have good erections even though there may be some pain with them, oral treatment with L-arginine and pentoxifylline may be used. As mentioned earlier, these agents seem to have an antiscarring effect and in time, clinical studies may prove them to be truly beneficial. At this point they appear to be the most promising oral agents.

If you have mild to moderate disease (less than 45 degrees), the recommended treatment may include the same oral drugs—L-arginine and pentoxifylline—as well as iontophoresis (EMDA) with a combination of verapamil and dexamethasone. Periodic vacuum therapy or daily external traction therapy may also be recommended.

If you want the most aggressive approach short of surgery regardless of your deformity, a three-armed approach is recommended. This includes oral treatment with daily Viagra, Cialis, or Levitra in addition to L-arginine and pentoxifylline, intralesional injection of verapamil once every two weeks, and daily use of an external penile traction device. This combination of medical therapy (which encourages chemical changes) and stretching therapy (which uses mechanical forces) may provide the best opportunity for improvement without surgery.

2. If I'm experiencing pain, are there any nonsurgical treatments, or combination of treatments, that I should avoid?

Vacuum therapy is not advised when the disease process is active and there is pain as this can stretch nerve fibers, resulting in more pain. Therefore, vacuum therapy without additional medical treatment, such as intralesional verapamil injections, is not advised in the acute phase of Peyronie's disease, particularly when there is significant pain.

3. Are all the non-surgical treatments discussed in this book available at all medical centers and urology offices?

At this time, there are a limited number of centers offering the full spectrum of Peyronie's disease treatments, including nonsurgical therapy and surgery. This is because, historically, physician training in Peyronie's disease has been limited. Fortunately, that's changing. The number of medical schools and teaching hospitals offering training in Peyronie's disease to their urology students/residents is growing rapidly. Thanks to better educational programs, new textbooks on Peyronie's disease, and new research providing insights into the cause and treatment of Peyronie's disease, it is hopeful that more urologists will take an interest in this disease and offer a complete range of treatment.

In the meantime, if you are seeking more advanced treatment of Peyronie's disease, such as intralesional injection therapy, iontophoresis, or surgery, it is best to discuss this with your primary care physician or your local urologist to determine their familiarity with the problem. If these physicians don't have experience with treating Peyronie's disease, or if they are not aware of or are not capable of offering the treatments, then pursuing a recognized expert in Peyronie's disease would be advised.

4. Are nonsurgical treatments for Peyronie's disease covered by insurance?

It depends. Most insurance companies will cover an initial evaluation, but some will not cover what they call "experimental" treatments. Typically, iontophoresis is covered, but the reimbursement rate is quite poor. Intralesional injection therapy is typically covered by insurance. External stretching tools, such as vacuum devices, are typically covered by insurance to some degree, but external penile extender devices are not covered.

When nonsurgical treatments are not covered by your medical insurance, the price varies from inexpensive oral medications to around $250 to $500 for an external vacuum device, $300 for an external penile extender, $1,200 for a complete iontophoresis setup, and $250-$300 per intralesional injection.

Part III

Surgical Treatment

9

Plication Procedures

Surgery is considered the gold standard of treatment to reduce penile curvature and improve sexual function. If nonsurgical treatments haven't provided you with satisfactory results, surgery may be an option for you. Of course, the idea of having surgery on your penis may be a little frightening. That's understandable, but you should know that the majority of men who have penile surgery are satisfied with the results.

There are three types of operations that treat Peyronie's disease: plication, excision and grafting, and the insertion of a prosthesis. Plication and grafting correct penile deformity, and a penile prosthesis corrects both deformity and erectile dysfunction. The operation that's right for you depends on the severity of your penile deformity and whether or not you have erectile dysfunction. Your doctor will determine which operation is best for you.

1. What is the goal of penile straightening surgery? If I have surgery, will my penis be like it was before I developed Peyronie's disease?

It is very important before delving into surgery that you understand the goals of penile straightening surgery, which are to make your penis functionally straight as well as to preserve your erectile rigidity. A functionally straight penis is defined as having a residual curve of less than 20 degrees, which should enable you to engage in sexual intercourse. In fact, most men can function quite well with curvature of less than 30 degrees in any direction. Unfortunately, no treatment at this time, either medical or surgical, can guarantee a recovery of your pre-Peyronie's disease penis.

2.   What is involved with plication procedure?

The surgical procedure *plication* is used to correct mild to moderate penile deformity due to Peyronie's disease. The least invasive surgical treatment of Peyronie's disease, plication involves shortening the "longer" side of the penis. For example, if the penis is curved in an upward direction towards your chin, then the longer side of the penis is on the undersurface. Therefore, to straighten the penis in this circumstance, tucks are made on the undersurface of the penis adjacent to the urethra.

All the surgical maneuvers take place under the skin, so there are no visible sutures or scars. The surgical procedure usually takes sixty to ninety minutes to perform.

3.   Are all plication operations the same?

Numerous techniques have been described to plicate the penis. The first plication operations were described by Dr. Reed Nesbit in the 1960s. In the Nesbit procedure, a portion of the outer jacket or tunic of the penis was actually excised to shorten the "longer" side. More recent modifications of Nesbit's operation do not fully expose the underlying vascular tissue in the hope that this would reduce the likelihood of postoperative erectile dysfunction.

Modern plication procedures use tucks rather than *excision* on the side of the penis that is opposite the direction of the curvature in order to shorten it so that both sides end up being equal, resulting in straightening. This is to say that if the penis were curved upward towards the belly, then the tucks would be positioned on the undersurface of the penis adjacent to the urethra. By shortening the urethral side, the penis will be straightened.

4. How do I know if I'm a candidate for plication surgery?

The best candidates for plication surgery have mild to moderate curvature of less than 60 to 70 degrees and can achieve an erection with satisfactory rigidity. If you have mild to moderate curvature and erectile dysfunction that responds to oral medication, you may be eligible for a plication operation. Plication surgery does not correct indentation or narrowing, conditions that can result in a *hinge-effect* or buckling of the penis. If severe indentation or narrowing are not corrected, the penis may be straight but unstable during sex. Therefore, a plication procedure is best performed when there is no significant indentation or narrowing. Your physician will determine if plication surgery is right for you.

5. Do I need to do anything special before having plication surgery? Should I stop having sex or stop taking any medications?

You do not need to abstain from having sex prior to plication surgery, but you should avoid certain medications that could increase the chances of postoperative bleeding. These include aspirin, Vitamin E, blood thinners such as Coumadin and Plavix, and herbs such as ginseng and gingko biloba. Your physician will provide you with details on when you should stop taking these drugs.

6. Do plication procedures require a hospital stay or anesthesia?

Plication operations are generally performed on an outpatient basis, meaning that you will go home the same day as your surgery. No overnight hospital stay is necessary. Anesthesia is used for the procedure, and your doctor may choose to use general anesthesia, regional anesthesia, local anesthesia, sedation, or some combination thereof.

General anesthesia renders you unconscious and blocks your memory of the procedure. Basically, you won't see, hear, or feel anything during your procedure. General anesthesia agents remain in the body for up to twenty-four hours, and you won't feel like you're back to normal until it has been completely eliminated from your system.

Regional anesthesia blocks sensation in a particular region of your body. For a plication procedure, this would be the lower half of the body. With regional anesthesia, you remain awake. However, it may be used in conjunction with sedation, so you may not remember the procedure.

Local anesthesia numbs a small portion of your body so you won't feel any pain in that area. When local anesthesia is used alone, you are fully awake and alert. Local anesthesia is often combined with sedation, so you may have no memories of the procedure. Local anesthetics don't cause any feelings of sleepiness or grogginess as they only remain in your system for a short time.

Sedation anesthesia, which uses a combination of sedatives and pain relievers, is often combined with regional or local anesthetics to induce relaxation and to provide additional pain relief. With sedation anesthesia, you can expect to feel normal within a few hours after surgery because the drugs don't remain in the body for very long.

7.   Can any urologist perform a plication procedure?

The Nesbit procedure and other plication operations are less risky than other penile straightening surgeries, and therefore may be performed by any urologist who is comfortable with this technique. When choosing a surgeon for a plication operation, be sure to ask how often the surgeon performs the procedure. Although there is no specific number to look for, it's a good idea to choose a surgeon who performs the procedure on a regular basis.

Plication Procedure

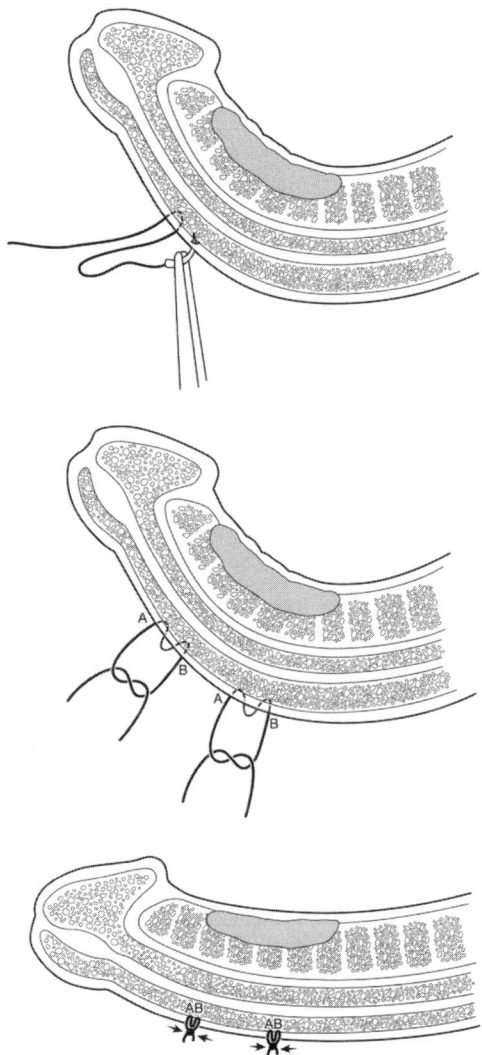

Mild cases of Peyronie's disease may be treated with plication, a surgical procedure in which the longer side of the penis is shortened in order to eliminate the curve.

8. Should I expect any pain after plication surgery?

Postoperative pain is generally mild, with most men taking nothing more than Tylenol. However, you may experience some pain at night due to nocturnal erections. This is a good thing—it shows that there's blood flow to the penis, that you're getting erections, and that the tissues are being stretched. If these nocturnal erections are very painful, your doctor can prescribe a pain medication.

9. Is there any kind of postoperative therapy I need to do following plication surgery? When can I resume sexual activity?

Approximately two weeks after surgery, your surgeon may recommend that you begin penile massage and stretching therapy twice a day for five minutes at a time for two weeks. During the next two weeks—weeks four through six after surgery—your surgeon may recommend that you have your partner perform the massage and stretching exercises. This is to help reintroduce your partner to touching your penis and to help your partner feel comfortable that they aren't going to injure your penis. You can resume sexual activity after approximately six weeks.

10. Are most patients who go through the plication procedure better off after the surgery than before?

Most of the current plication operations have a high rate of success. In fact, up to 99 percent experience satisfactory straightening and minimal compromise in erectile function. Again, by understanding the goals and limits of penile straightening surgery before you undergo the procedure, you are more likely to be satisfied with the results.

11. Does plication surgery cause a change in penile sexual sensation?

By and large the plication operation results in very little reported change in penile sexual sensation. The primary sensory nerves of the penis run on the top surface of the penis as you look down upon it. Therefore, if the curvature is upward towards your belly, the plications made to straighten the penis are performed on the undersurface of the penis adjacent to the urethra. There are very few nerves there and therefore significant loss of sensation is unlikely. On the other hand, if the curvature is downward or downward and lateral then it will require careful mobilization of the nerves on the surface of the penis to reduce the likelihood of postoperative reduced penile sexual sensation. Even in these operations the likelihood of substantial loss of sensation is extraordinarily rare and tends to recover with time, usually in about six to twelve months.

12. Do plication operations result in a shortening of the penis?

Plication operations can result in a shortening of the penis. A recent study demonstrated that the expected loss of length depends on the direction and degree of curvature. For example, men who have upward or lateral curvature tend to have very little loss of length (less than one half inch). In general, the less curvature you have, the less length you can expect to lose. For men with less than 60 degrees of curvature, loss of length is minimal. Men with severe curvature in excess of 70 degrees experience a greater loss of length, which is why plication is not recommended to correct severe curvature even if you can achieve erections with satisfactory rigidity.

13. What are the chances that plication will cause erectile dysfunction?

The plication operation is less invasive than the other surgeries for Peyronie's disease and therefore is the least likely to result in diminished rigidity. The modern plication procedures are designed to avoid injury to the underlying vascular tissue contained within the erectile bodies. Therefore, preservation of erectile function tends to be in the 95 percent or higher range. Further, plication does not interfere with the function of the urethra for urination and ejaculation.

14. I recently had penile plication surgery. I have no feeling in the last inch of the shaft and the head. Is this normal, and will the feeling return when I am further healed?

In some plication procedures, the sensory nerves supplying the shaft and the head of the penis may be moved or slightly damaged. These sensory nerves run on the top surface of the penis. Therefore, if you have a downward curve, it is likely that these nerves have to be mobilized. Typically, when nerves are moved or slightly damaged, there will be a period of numbness, which will go away over time. Nerves heal very slowly and it may take three to twelve months to recover complete sensation. If the nerves were completely damaged, then the likelihood of complete recovery of nerve sensation is reduced. However, you may still be able to achieve satisfactory sexual sensation. This is because nerves from other areas of the penis can grow into the damaged area.

15. What are the side effects associated with penile surgery?

Although surgery is considered the gold standard for the correction of penile deformity, there are potential side effects to surgery. Older studies on surgery for Peyronie's disease suggested that there may be a very high rate of erectile dysfunction and recurrence of deformity as well as loss of sensation. Fortunately, more recent studies have demonstrated much better results.

When surgery is performed by an experienced surgeon, side effects occur infrequently but may include incomplete straightening, recurrent curvature, shortening of the penis, diminished sensation, delayed ejaculation, or erectile dysfunction. For the men who develop some erectile dysfunction after surgery, most are not completely impotent, but may notice that they require medicines like Viagra, Cialis, or Levitra in order to obtain and/or sustain a good erection. These problems do not happen commonly, and they certainly happen less often when the physician performs these operations regularly.

10

Surgical Grafting

Grafting is a surgical procedure that is used to correct severe penile deformity due to Peyronie's disease. In this operation, small incisions are made in the Peyronie's plaque, or in some cases small portions of the plaque are actually removed. This is done in an effort to lengthen the portion of the penis that has been shortened due to the scar.

Any incisions made in the plaque or any areas of the plaque that have been removed need to be covered with grafts to help keep blood trapped within the cylinders of the penis, something that is necessary in order to achieve an erection.

1. What are surgical grafts and where do they come from?

Grafts are small pieces of soft tissue that are used to cover the incisions made in the plaque. There are many different types of grafts that can be used for this procedure. The newest approach for grafting the penis uses "off-the-shelf" grafts. These grafts are typically made from human cadaver tissue or animal tissue that has been processed to remove all cellular material, bacteria, and viral elements leaving behind a collagen matrix upon which your own tissue will grow over a twelve- to eighteen-month period. The human cadaver tissue typically comes from the pericardium, a sac that encloses the heart. Animal grafts are often made from pig intestines and are referred to as SIS, or *small intestinal submucosa.*

Grafts can also be taken from another area of your body. Grafts that come from your own body are called *autologous.* These grafts have been harvested from fat, skin, vein (typically taken from the leg), *temporalis fascia* (a thick flat piece of tissue found under the skin behind the ear), or the *tunica vaginalis* (a tissue found within the *scrotum* surrounding the testicle). Even flaps of skin mobilized from the foreskin have been used successfully.

Some doctors still use vein grafts due to their belief that since the outer jacket of the penis is a blood-containing structure, a vein is a suitable grafting material. Other autologous grafts aren't used as commonly as they once were. In fact, fat, skin, and tunica vaginalis grafts are rarely used anymore. The results with tunica vaginalis grafting have not been particularly successful in that the graft tends to contract.

In the past, various synthetic grafts were used, including patches made of Dacron, silicone, or Gore-Tex. The synthetic grafts are not recommended at all now as they typically remain palpable, and if they become infected, it is a much more complicated operation to remove them.

Note: I have not used a tunica vaginalis graft in more than ten years because at least 50 percent of my previous tunica vaginalis grafts contracted so severely that the curvature recurred postoperatively.

2.   What are the advantages and disadvantages of the various types of grafts?

Off-the-shelf grafts have two big advantages: they shorten operating time by an hour or more, and using them means you won't have to have a secondary incision in your body to harvest a graft. There are some drawbacks associated with using an autogolgus graft. It increases the length of time you'll need to spend in the operating room; it requires additional incisions in your body; and there's a risk for complications associated with the additional wound. In addition, with vein grafts, the vein that is typically used is the same vein that is used in bypass surgeries. In a hypothetical situation, if you have a vein graft for repairing the penis and then someday need heart bypass surgery, you wouldn't have that vein available.

3. Does the whole plaque need to be removed?

Historically, surgeons believed that the Peyronie's plaque was the sole representation of the disease and therefore it was felt that the entire scar had to be removed during a grafting operation to get successful straightening and a low recurrence rate. Over the past decade, it has been recognized that a less invasive operation may result in equal correction of deformity, and cause less erectile dysfunction than with full plaque excision and grafting. This is because with the incision or partial excision there is not as much exposure of the erectile tissue and therefore the scarring or injury to this tissue is diminished. When total plaque excision was performed, up to 20 to 80 percent of men developed erectile dysfunction postoperatively. Today, with the incision or partial excision procedure, that percentage is much lower.

4. How do I know if I'm a candidate for grafting surgery?

Grafting surgery is reserved for those who have severe deformity but are still able to achieve a good-quality erection. In terms of grafting surgery, severe deformity is defined as having curvature that exceeds 70 degrees and/or having substantial narrowing or indentation that has resulted in an unstable penis that buckles or has a hinge-effect, making intercourse quite difficult and occasionally painful.

To be considered a good candidate for grafting surgery, you must be able to achieve good-quality erections in spite of the deformity. Being able to achieve an erection with excellent quality rigidity is very important because this procedure has a higher risk for postoperative erectile dysfunction than the plication procedure. Ask yourself, "If my penis were straight, and there were no curvature or indentation, would the hardness of the erection that I currently experience be adequate for sexual activity?" If the answer to this question is a resounding "Yes," then you may be a candidate for the grafting procedure. One group of men who might truly benefit from the grafting operation would be those who have a substantially shortened penis, where any further shortening that may occur with a plication operation would not be acceptable.

5. Why does grafting surgery have a higher risk for postoperative erectile dysfunction than plication surgery?

The incisions made in the plaque or the partial excision of the plaque during a grafting operation results in the opening of the *tunica albuginea*, the outer jacket of the penis that covers the erectile cylinders; this exposes the underlying vascular tissue and makes it vulnerable to injury. Because of this, there is an increased risk of postoperative erectile dysfunction. Erectile dysfunction is thought to be a result of exposure and injury to the underlying erectile vascular tissue. This results in either inadequate inward flow of blood to fill the penis properly or in an inadequate expansion of the erectile tissue, and a *venous leak* occurs. When a venous leak occurs, the blood runs into the penis and then runs out, preventing a full, rigid erection.

Studies on men who would be most at risk for developing erectile dysfunction following a grafting procedure show that the quality of erectile function prior to surgery can help predict postoperative results. This means that if you have some compromise to your erections preoperatively, you are not likely to get better and may get worse.

Reports show that the rate of erectile dysfunction is minimal and in the 5 to 15 percent range in men who have good-quality erections before surgery or who can achieve good-quality erections using oral erection medications, such as Viagra, Levitra, or Cialis. Most men who experience postoperative ED will respond to the use of oral erection medications after surgery. But there is the possibility of more severe ED, which would require more advanced treatment including vacuum therapy, injection therapy, or intraurethral suppositories (MUSE). With

Surgical Scar Removal with Grafting

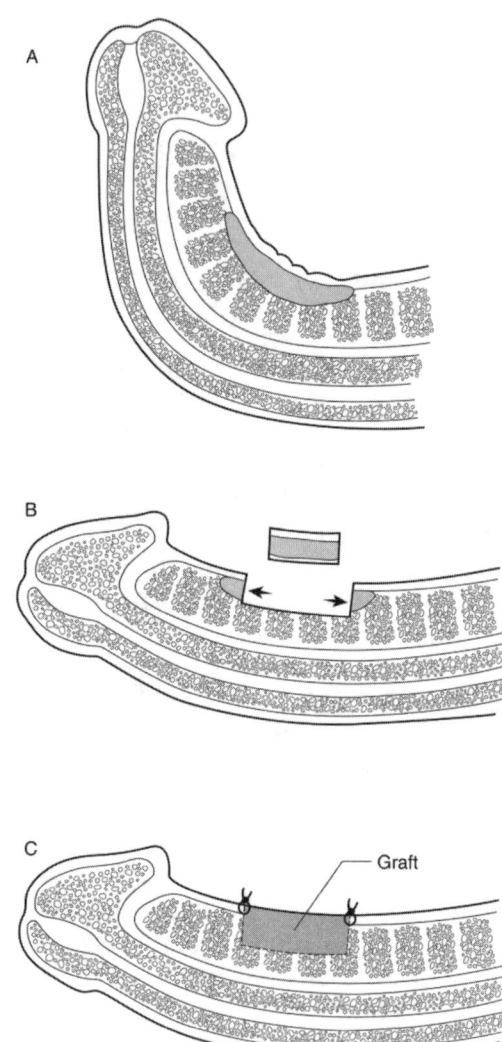

More severe deformities can be treated with surgical removal of the scar tissue. A variety of grafts are used to replace the skin removed.

MUSE a tiny pellet containing erection drugs is inserted into the urethra using a slender applicator.

It is extremely rare to see complete and permanent erectile dysfunction following a grafting procedure in a man who has good-quality erections preoperatively, especially when the procedure is performed by an expert in penile reconstruction for Peyronie's disease. Should severe ED occur, there is still hope. A penile prosthesis may be placed at a later time and will not be compromised by the prior grafting operation.

6.   If I have some erectile dysfunction prior to grafting surgery, what are the likely results? Will grafting surgery prevent me from being able to have a penile prosthesis at a later date?

Men who have mild to moderate erectile dysfunction and who have less than complete responses to oral erection drugs should know that grafting surgery will not improve the erectile dysfunction and may actually make it worse. However, you should be aware that if you elect to undergo the grafting procedure and you develop severe ED after surgery, a penile prosthesis may be implanted in a subsequent operation without difficulty. That some men simply will not accept a penile prosthesis without first trying the grafting operation is totally reasonable, but they must fully understand the potential risks.

7.   Can any urologist perform grafting surgery?

Grafting is a delicate surgery that requires experienced hands. Because there's a higher risk for postoperative erectile dysfunction with this procedure, make sure you choose your surgeon carefully. If you're considering grafting surgery, it's advisable to go to an expert in the field of penile reconstruction for Peyronie's disease. If your doctor is not an expert in this field, you may want to ask for a recommendation. You can also search for a Peyronie's specialist in your area at www.peyroniesassociation.org.

8. Do I need to do anything special to prepare for grafting surgery, such as abstaining from sex or avoiding any medications?

There's no reason why you would need to abstain from sexual activity prior to grafting surgery provided that the severity of your deformity doesn't limit your ability to achieve penetration. As for medications, you should avoid anything that could increase post-operative bleeding, including aspirin, Vitamin E, blood-thinning drugs like Coumadin and Plavix, as well as herbs such as ginseng and gingko biloba. If you are taking any other medications or over-the-counter vitamins or herbs, you should ask your doctor if you should stop taking them prior to surgery.

9. Do grafting procedures require a hospital stay or anesthesia?

Grafting procedures take from two and a half to four hours to perform and are typically outpatient procedures, meaning that you will go home the same day as your surgery. Anesthesia is used for the procedure, and your doctor may choose to use general anesthesia, regional anesthesia, local anesthesia, sedation, or some combination thereof.

10. What will the recovery period after grafting surgery be like? Is it painful? Do I need to do any postoperative therapy?

The recovery period following grafting surgery is very similar to what is experienced after a plication procedure. As with plication, pain following grafting surgery is usually minimal and most men get by with nothing more than Tylenol. In some cases, pain may be experienced with nocturnal erections. These nighttime erections are a good sign that your penis is getting blood flow, that you're achieving erections, and that the tissues are being stretched. If nocturnal erections are very painful, your doctor can prescribe medication to alleviate the pain.

Your surgeon may recommend the same postoperative therapy that is advised following plication surgery. Penile massage and stretching therapy should begin about two weeks after your procedure and should be performed twice a day for five minutes at a time for two weeks. Your doctor may recommend having your partner perform the massage and stretching exercises during weeks four through six after surgery. This is to alleviate any fears that they will injure your penis when touching it. Sexual activity can resume after approximately six weeks.

11. Do grafting operations make the penis longer?

By and large, the grafting operation will make the constricted, shortened side of the penis equal to the opposite side, thereby making the penis straight. If the penis is curved upward, which is the most common deformity, the incision is made through the scar on the top surface of the penis in order to lengthen this side of the penis. This may result in some increased length of the penis from the pubic bone to the tip of the penis.

Reports show that up to 70 percent of men may note anywhere from a one-half inch to one inch increase in length, but 30 percent may note some shortening. The cause of the shortening is not clear, but it is thought that it may be due to the generalized loss of elasticity that occurs in the penile tissues in men with Peyronie's disease. Regardless, the loss of length tends to be small at one-quarter to one-half inch and is not typically compromising. Overall, the risk of penile shortening is much less with the grafting procedure than with the plication procedure.

12. Does grafting cause any side effects?

Erectile dysfunction is the most recognized and potentially most disturbing complication following the incision or partial excision and grafting procedure. There are also other complications or side effects from this operation that need to be fully understood by the patient.

They include incomplete straightening, change in penile sensation, delayed ejaculation, and recurrent curvature, although this is rare if surgery is performed when the disease has already reached the stable stage. In the properly selected patient and in the hands of an experienced surgeon, the likelihood of any of these complications being severe or permanent is low and in the 5 to 10 percent range.

13. Do grafting operations cause a change in penile sensation?

Grafting operations, when performed by experts in the field, rarely cause any permanent loss of sensation. However, it is not uncommon for the first several days to months after surgery to experience a change in sensation. You may experience diminished sensation or a sense of numbness, or may experience hypersensitivity of the penis. The key here is that it is rare for these changes to be permanent, and a period of sexual rehabilitation after surgery is always advisable to encourage nerve recovery.

The most common change reported may be a diminished appreciation of sexual arousal, which may result in some delayed ejaculation and orgasm. Some men have found this to be a benefit as it can eradicate problems of premature ejaculation. It is important for the prospective patient who is undergoing this operation to understand that this may occur and that it typically improves with time.

The reason changes in sensation occur is that to get to the plaque, it is usually necessary to elevate the nerves and blood vessels that run over the surface of the penis and directly over the plaque. Mobilization of this tissue, when done without care, may result in diminished penile sensitivity or even numbness. This is rarely the case with an experienced urologic reconstructive surgeon.

11

Prosthesis Implantation

penile prosthesis is a device that is placed within the penis to correct erectile dysfunction. The prosthesis consists of a pair of fluid-filled inflatable cylinders and a pump. The cylinders, which are tubular and run the length of the penis, are implanted inside the penis. The pump, which is about the size of your thumb, is placed within the scrotum. The pump is connected to the cylinders by tubing. By squeezing on the pump, the cylinders will inflate, causing the penis to become rigid. These devices result in excellent rigidity with a high rate of mechanical reliability and a low rate of infection, less than 2 percent.

1. How is the penile prosthesis procedure performed?

During penile prothesis surgery, the surgeon makes a small opening in the scrotal sac, which allows for placement of the prosthesis in the penis and for placement of the pump in the scrotum. It is a relatively minor procedure that takes one to two hours to perform.

2. Is the deformity from Peyronie's disease corrected during the procedure?

During the procedure, a straightening technique known as manual modeling is performed to correct the deformity. To perform manual modeling, the surgeon will inflate the prosthesis that has just been placed in the penis to see the penile curvature. The surgeon will then bend the penis in the opposite way of the curvature and keep it bent for thirty to sixty seconds in an attempt to stretch the scar tissue. This bending of the penis is performed repeatedly until functional straightening—30 degrees or less—is achieved. The correction achieved using this technique is permanent. In addition, any residual curvature will continue to improve over the next six months with use of the prosthesis because it acts as an internal stretching device.

3. Who is a good candidate for a penile prosthesis?

If you have significant erectile insufficiency, or you cannot obtain or maintain a good erection when sexually aroused, you may benefit from the placement of an inflatable penile prosthesis. Prosthesis placement can be performed whether you have mild, moderate, or severe deformity. Success rates with this approach have been excellent in terms of straightening and result in a rigid penis for intercourse on demand. The best candidates for penile prosthesis placement and manual modeling include men who are older and/or who have a history of vascular disease, frequently due to diabetes, high blood pressure, elevated cholesterol, or a long history of smoking, either currently or in the past.

4. Should I avoid any medications prior to penile prosthesis surgery?

Similar to plication and grafting procedures, you should avoid anything that could increase postoperative bleeding, including aspirin, Vitamin E, blood-thinning drugs like Coumadin or Plavix, and herbs such as ginseng and gingko biloba. If you are taking any other medications or over-the-counter vitamins or herbs, you should ask your doctor if you should stop taking them prior to surgery.

5. Does penile prosthesis surgery require a hospital stay or anesthesia?

There is no hospital stay required for a penile prosthesis procedure, but the outpatient procedure does require anesthesia. General anesthesia or regional anesthesia are commonly used for these procedures.

6. What is the recovery period like? Is it normal to experience pain after the surgery?

Following surgery, significant swelling can occur, which will stretch the nerves inside the penis and result in pain. Pain after surgery varies and is highly individual; some men have very little pain, but most have a lot for seven to fourteen days. Typically, after the first two weeks, the pain level diminishes markedly and by six to ten weeks, the pain is usually gone. Your doctor can recommend over-the-counter pain relievers or can give you a prescription for pain medication if necessary.

7. Is there any postoperative therapy I need to perform? When can I have sex again?

Your surgeon will likely recommend that you begin postoperative therapy approximately one month after your surgery. Very simply, you'll be asked to begin cycling the prosthesis — inflating it and deflating it — twice a day. Around this same time, at about four to six weeks after surgery, you can resume sexual activity.

8. Are all penile prostheses the same?

There are inflatable prostheses and noninflatable prostheses. For men with Peyronie's disease, inflatable prostheses are always recommended. Noninflatable prostheses are bendable and can be manipulated to achieve an erection. These devices typically result in an unnatural appearance as the penis is always hard. Placement of a noninflatable prosthesis is not recommended if you have Peyronie's disease because these devices do not correct the deformity as well as an inflatable prosthesis does. Inflatable prostheses within the penis act as internal tissue expanders and can correct residual curvature postoperatively over a six to twelve month period.

9. What are the reported satisfaction rates for inflatable penile prostheses in men with Peyronie's disease?

The satisfaction rates of patients with Peyronie's disease receiving an inflatable prosthesis have appeared to be slightly less than that of patients with penile prostheses who do not have Peyronie's disease. This may be reflective of the psychological distress caused by this disorder. However, mechanical failure rates and infection rates are no higher in patients with Peyronie's disease. As a result, the few published studies on satisfaction rates report that 80 to 90 percent of men with Peyronie's disease are satisfied with their inflatable prostheses with respect to ease of operation, concealability, and naturalness of the erection.

10. Do inflatable penile prostheses change penile sensation, ejaculation, or orgasm?

If you have ED and Peyronie's disease, and you're capable of experiencing ejaculation and orgasm in a less than fully rigid state, then you shouldn't expect any changes in regard to sensation, ejaculation, or orgasm. The prosthesis will not change that. Therefore, if you cannot experience an ejaculation or orgasm without an erect penis, the prosthesis can now provide the needed hardness.

As men age, with or without PD, it's common to experience a reduced power of ejaculation and diminished intensity of orgasm. This may be due to a generalized loss of sensation or sexual enthusiasm, and the prosthesis may not correct these issues. In some cases, the sensation of the penis may be slightly diminished. This may result in a prolonged time to experience orgasm.

Manual Straightening
during Prothesis Insertion

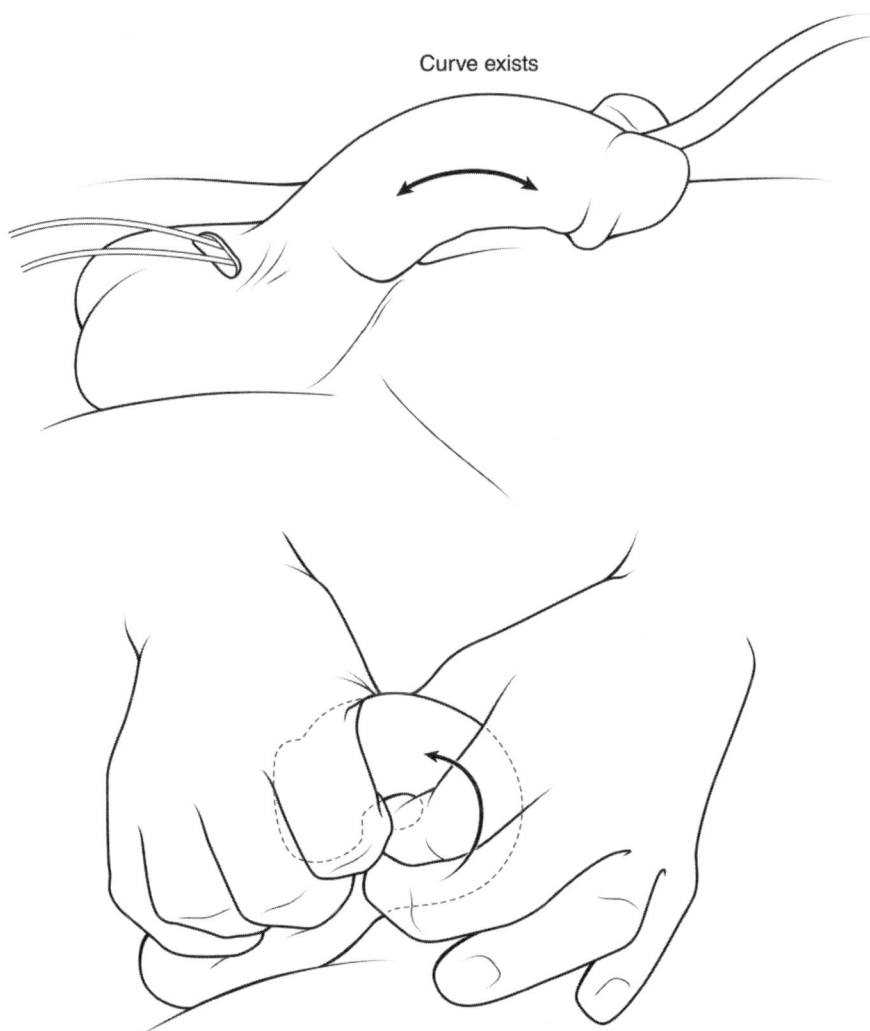

Curve exists

During the implantation of the prosthesis, the surgeon performs manual modeling to straighten the penis. Once the prosthesis in place, the surgeon bends the penis to stretch the scar tissue; the improvement gained is permanent.

It is important to note that the prosthesis allows for the rapid development of an erection whether you are sexually aroused or not. Therefore, if you develop an erection as a result of pumping the prosthesis, but you aren't yet psychologically aroused, it may take some time for orgasm to occur. With time, you'll likely adjust to this. There will always be some period of adjustment to the presence of the prosthesis for both you and your partner.

11. Do inflatable penile prostheses interfere with urination?

No. These devices are placed in the erectile bodies, which are the paired vascular cylinders within the penis. These are separate from the urethra, which is the structure that carries the *semen* and urine out of the penis. Therefore, you should not experience any changes in urination.

12. Will the penile prosthesis look natural? Will I feel it all the time? Are there any other changes to my body I should be aware of?

Initially, following surgery, it's common to experience some partial rigidity, which may make it difficult to conceal the device. This improves with time as healing and tissue softening occurs. It may take 2 to 6 months for the appearance of the penis to become "natural" and for it to be readily concealed, particularly in the flaccid state under clothing. Once you're completely healed, a well-placed prosthesis should not be apparent. These are completely internal devices. The pumps that are placed within the scrotum, when positioned properly, are not apparent either. One misconception that needs to be clarified is that, contrary to popular belief, there is typically no visible evidence of the surgery on the shaft of the penis.

Likewise, once the healing process is complete, you won't be aware of the presence of the prosthesis. The initial stage after surgery can be quite painful, but this will simply resolve with time. Once the

Penile Prothesis

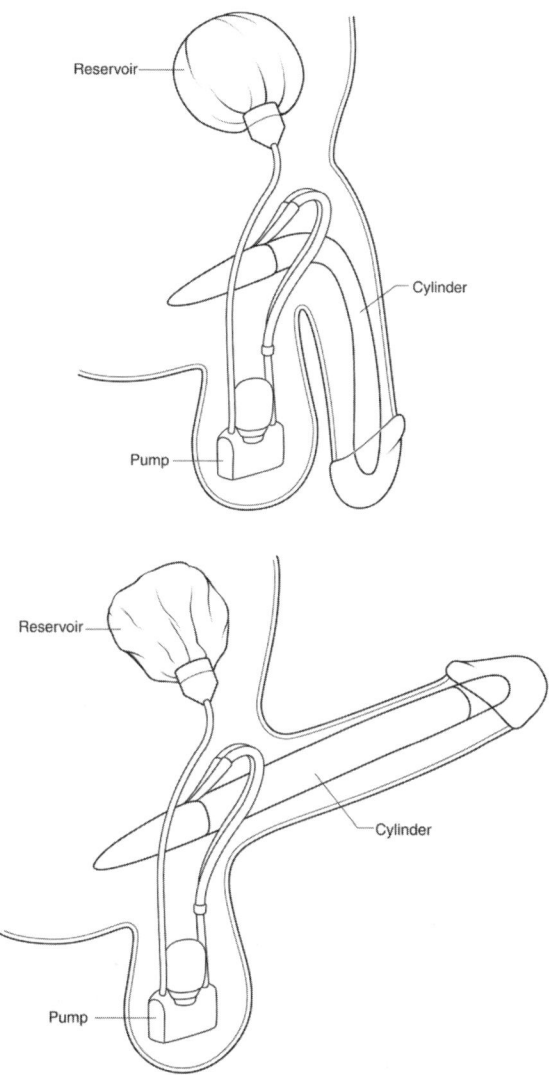

The top illustration shows the prosthesis in a flaccid penis. The lower illustration shows the inflated prosthesis. The device has three parts: the paired cylinders inside the penis, the pump in the scrotum, and the reservoir, which holds a saline solution, behind the abdominal muscles.

pain does disappear, the presence of the prosthesis is similar to a wrist-watch. Typically, you are not aware of the watch unless you touch it. Similarly, you will not be aware that the prosthesis is in your body unless you touch it directly.

Penile prostheses are designed for one purpose, and that is to provide rigidity when you want it, as long as you want it, and whenever you want it. They should not cause any other changes to your body and they do not interfere with urination, ejaculation, orgasm, or sexual sensation.

13. Will my sexual partner be able to see or feel the penile prosthesis?

Typically, a sexual partner will not notice a prosthesis. The pump is smaller than a testicle and the cylinders are soft and barely palpable in the flaccid state. When the penis is erect, it typically looks and feels like a natural erection.

Note: I've had several young patients who did not respond to medical therapy for ED who had penile prostheses placed. These prostheses were placed before these men were married, and they elected not to tell their girlfriends or future wives that they had a prosthesis. Apparently the women did not know that the device was present.

14. Will I feel like a mechanical man because I have a penile prosthesis?

There is a period of adjustment to having a penile prosthesis. This includes the healing process during which there can be pain and swelling. This period typically takes less than two to three months after surgery, and then things look pretty natural. There is also a period of adjustment in learning how to inflate it and deflate it which, in time, can be done almost unconsciously. The final adjustment is recognizing that when you have interest in sexual activity, and you have that sense of sexual arousal in your mind and body, that inflation of the prosthesis will guarantee a fully rigid penis. It is at this point that normal sexual activity can be achieved and enjoyed.

It should also be recognized that the prosthesis can be inflated in the non-aroused state and in this circumstance, it may take quite a bit longer to reach orgasm because you are not starting out sexually aroused. Therefore, the bottom line is that the prosthesis is designed to provide rigidity only; all the rest comes from you and your interaction with your partner.

15. My partner says she does not want me to have a penile prosthesis because she is concerned that the erection that I get is not due to her stimulating me. How do I handle this?

This type of thinking can interfere with success after placement of the prosthesis. If you find your female partner is resistant to the idea of a penile prosthesis, this needs to be addressed with your doctor or possibly even with a sex therapist. When you become sexually aroused and want to engage in sexual intercourse but cannot because of poor-quality erection, you'll need the prosthesis to create the needed rigidity. The emotions involved in terms of the level of the intimacy and the lovemaking itself is between you and your partner.

16. Can I expect that my penis will be bigger as a result of having a prosthesis?

The penis will not be any longer as a result of placement of the prosthesis, it will only be able to become rigid when it is inflated. It seems that virtually all men want a larger penis. This remains somewhat of a male mystery. Unfortunately, with Peyronie's disease, there is often-times shaft shortening as well as a loss of girth as a result of the scarring process preventing expansion of the outer jacket. The prostheses are designed to fill the space within the tunica albuginea that is normally filled with the vascular tissue. The prosthesis will fill the space when it is inflated and expand the tunica albuginea to its maximum capacity.

Recent studies have examined patients before and after surgery to see if any shortening occurs as a result of placement of a prosthesis. By and large, when properly fitted, shortening tends to be negligible, approximately half an inch. This is typically not a noticeable amount. The best way to assess the length that you might obtain with a penile prosthesis is to grasp the head/glans of the penis and pull it straight away from your body at a right angle (toward the ceiling when lying on your back). The maximum stretch will be the length of the penis with a properly placed prosthesis.

It should also be recognized that the penile prosthesis fills the *corpora cavernosa*, the cylinders that contain the vascular tissue, which provides support for the head/glans of the penis but does not cause it to become engorged with blood with sexual stimulation. If your glans becomes engorged when sexually aroused before the placement of the prosthesis, it should continue to do so after placement of a prosthesis. This will give the appearance of a natural erection. On the other hand, if your vascular disease is so significant that the head/glans does not fill when sexually stimulated, the prosthesis will support the head of the penis, but you will not get the engorgement.

The girth of the penis is also limited to some degree by the expansion of the tunica albuginea and is somewhat dependent upon the nature of the device used. If the Peyronie's process has caused signif- icant circumferential scarring, this may result in persistent narrowing after the operation. But modern-day penile prostheses seem to have such good rigidity that they may act as tissue expanders and result in some increase in girth over time.

17. Once I have placement of a penile prosthesis, how long can I expect it to work?

These devices are designed to work for life, but like any product that is placed within the body, such as an artificial knee or hip, a penile prosthesis may also fail from wear. The improvements in penile prosthesis design have markedly lowered the mechanical failure rate.

Still, any device may fail, at any time, after placement. There are not many studies examining the life expectancy of penile prostheses beyond ten years. Most of the recent studies have suggested a 10 percent mechanical failure rate in ten years. Looking at the flip side, this means that 90 percent of patients should have a functional prosthesis ten years after it is implanted.

Most mechanical failures are due to a crack in the tubing or the cylinders, which leads to a leak of fluid. If your prosthesis were to fail mechanically, the fluid that is in the prosthesis—usually a saline solution, which is much like intravenous fluid—will be reabsorbed by your body and will not cause any harm whatsoever. If you are interested in continuing to be sexually active, another operation will be necessary to remove the defective component, or the entire device, and then replace it. This secondary operation tends to be much easier on you, as far as postoperative pain, because the space within the penis has already been created, resulting in much less postoperative inflammation, which is what leads to swelling and pain.

18. If my prosthesis fails mechanically, will I need to pay for a second operation?

Both of the companies distributing these devices in the U.S. offer lifetime warranties. This means that if the device were to fail mechanically, the cost of a new prosthesis would be covered by the manufacturer. Take note that this does not cover the costs for the surgical facility or the surgeon. You or your insurance company will be responsible for these costs.

19. What if my penile prosthesis becomes infected?

Penile prosthesis infections following surgery are rare, and studies show that infection occurs in only 0.5 to 1.5 percent of patients. This includes men who have undergone kidney, liver, and pancreas transplants; severe diabetics; and other immuno-suppressed individuals. The low rate of infections is due in part to the fact that both of the companies in the United States that manufacture inflatable penile prostheses use a special coating on the devices that tends to reduce the likelihood of infection. A key to avoiding infection is to go to an experienced surgeon who has a well-tuned program for penile prosthesis implantation and who has a low rate of reported infection.

Although rare, penile prosthesis infection is the most serious complication occurring with this operation. If an infection does occur, it is rare that the infection will be cured by the use of oral or intravenous antibiotics alone; an operation will be necessary to remove the entire device and replace it. It is critical to replace the prosthesis under the best possible circumstances. This means that the operating surgeon will typically use a variety of antibiotics before the incision is made, will bathe the tissues of the penis during the operation with antibiotics, and will send you home with oral antibiotics, all of which are used to reduce the likelihood of another postoperative infection. These "salvage" operations have been successful in up to 85 percent of cases.

20. Is penile prosthesis surgery always the best option for men over fifty?

If you have some erectile dysfunction, but you respond adequately to oral erection medications such as Viagra, Levitra, and Cialis, then you should consider surgical penile straightening without a prosthesis. If you're concerned about developing ED in the future, particularly if you have diabetes, high blood pressure, and/or a significant smoking history, then placement of a prosthesis may be the best option as it will solve the ED and PD problems.

Note: It is my opinion that if a man does not have significant ED, he does not need a prosthesis. Others have suggested that any man over the age of fifty with Peyronie's disease should have a prosthesis placed. I believe that this is too simple an answer and results in an irreversible change in the penis. Once the prosthesis is placed, you are forever dependent upon the internal device to develop good rigidity.

12

Common Questions
about Surgical Procedures

1. What are the side effects associated with penile surgery?

Although surgery is considered the gold standard for the correction of penile deformity, there are potential side effects to surgery. Older studies on surgery for Peyronie's disease suggested that there may be a very high rate of erectile dysfunction and recurrence of deformity as well as loss of sensation. Fortunately, more recent studies have demonstrated much better results.

When surgery is performed by an experienced surgeon, side effects occur infrequently but may include incomplete straightening, recurrent curvature, shortening of the penis, diminished sensation, delayed ejaculation, or erectile dysfunction. For the men who develop some erectile dysfunction after surgery, most are not completely impotent, but may notice that they require medicines like Viagra, Cialis, or Levitra in order to obtain and/or sustain a good erection. These problems do not happen commonly, and they certainly happen less often when the physician performs these operations regularly.

2. Are surgical procedures for Peyronie's disease covered by insurance?

All three of the surgical procedures to correct Peyronie's disease—plication, grafting, and prothesis placement—are typically covered by insurance when the surgery is medically indicated by a doctor. However, you should be aware that surgery can cost many thousands of dollars, and the amount covered depends on your insurance company and on your particular plan. Most of these surgical procedures can now be performed on an outpatient basis, which can substantially reduce the cost to you and/or your insurance company.

3. When can I have surgery to straighten my penis?

Surgery should only be recommended when the disease is stable. This means that there has been no significant change in the deformity and plaque configuration for at least six to nine months. In addition, any pain with the development of an erection or with direct touching of the penis should be gone. Most physicians recommend not offering surgery until at least one year after onset of the disease. Therefore, if you have a rapid development of deformity and then it stabilizes quickly, it is still best to wait a minimum of six to twelve months to ensure that the disease process is not going to recur after undergoing surgery.

4. Who should do the penile surgery to straighten my penis?

If you're considering undergoing reconstructive surgery on the penis, it is clearly an extremely important operation for you and you should choose your surgeon carefully. It is critical for the surgeon to have significant experience and training with these procedures, particularly when grafting is performed. The less complicated operations—plication and placement of a penile prosthesis with manual modeling—also require an experienced surgeon, but there are more urologic surgeons capable of performing these two operations. Plaque incision or partial excision and grafting, which is utilized for the most advanced deformities in men who have good erections before surgery, should only be performed by surgeons who are very experienced with this operation.

The best way to determine whether your surgeon is familiar with the operative techniques for men with Peyronie's disease is to ask them directly. The web site of the Association of Peyronie's Disease Advocates, www.peyroniesassociation.org, contains a list of doctors who are interested in Peyronie's disease and may be used as a resource.

5.   Which type of operation is best for me?

In general, the severity of your deformity and your ability or inability to achieve a good-quality erection will determine which procedure is best for you. Your doctor will base the decision largely on the tests performed during your evaluation. In addition, if you have significant calcification or bone formation, you are most likely a candidate for either a partial excision of the scar or placement of a prosthesis. When there is extensive calcification, medical therapy is usually of little value and surgery becomes the necessary approach.

In general, if you can achieve good-quality erections, you may be a candidate for penile straightening without a penile prosthesis. On the other hand, if there is insufficient erectile response even when taking medications like Viagra, Levitra, or Cialis, then penile prosthesis is recommended.

Lastly, when the decision is not absolutely clear before the operation, your surgeon may ask for permission to make the decision in the operating room, understanding that if the less complicated tunica plication can be performed, this would be preferred, but if the curvature-associated deformities are too severe, then incision and grafting will be done.

6.   What if I develop erectile dysfunction after surgery? What are my options?

It is possible for erectile dysfunction to occur after straightening surgery for Peyronie's disease. Before undergoing surgery, you should be evaluated for your erectile dysfunction to see if you respond to oral treatments such as Viagra, Levitra, or Cialis. If you aren't able to achieve a good-quality erection when using these drugs, then it may be advisable to have a penile prosthesis implanted while having the penis straightened at the same time. This is because men who have more advanced erectile dysfunction do not tend to recover their rigidity after surgery. In fact, the problem may become worse. If it does, it is still recommended that you again try Viagra, Levitra, and Cialis.

Other options include placing a suppository of blood vessel-dilating medicine known as MUSE into the urethra or using a vacuum constriction device. The goal of all of these treatments is to create a rigid penis that allows you to engage in sexual intercourse. Sexual arousal, pleasure, sensation, or ejaculation should not be significantly altered by any of these treatments.

If your postoperative erectile dysfunction doesn't respond to any of these approaches, or if you would prefer the most rapid and reliable way to obtain satisfactory rigidity, a penile prosthesis is recommended. A penile prosthesis can be readily placed as the straightening surgery does not interfere with the ability to place a prosthesis successfully.

7. I have a bend that goes straight down and slightly to the left. Would surgery help this type of Peyronie's?

This type of curvature is best treated with surgery. The type of surgery depends upon several factors. If Peyronie's disease has caused substantial shortening, or the penis is already short, then there is likely to be further shortening when correcting a downward curvature. The amount of shortening depends upon the degree of curvature. The more severe the curvature, the greater the amount of shortening. Studies have shown that the amount of length lost in men with curvature of less than 60 degrees tends to be the one-half-inch to three-quarter-inch range, but when curvature is in excess of 60 degrees, more shortening is possible.

On the other hand, if the curvature is severe (more than 70 degrees) and a grafting procedure is performed to correct it, there is a reported higher risk of erectile dysfunction, which approaches 50 percent of men undergoing grafting for downward curvature. Men with congenital downward curvature typically have increased elasticity and long penises. In these patients, a plication operation is usually recommended instead of a grafting procedure. This is because the degree of shortening in the man with congenital curvature tends to be less bothersome, and there is a substantially lower rate of postoperative erectile dysfunction with the plication procedure.

For men who have Peyronie's disease, severe downward curvature, and borderline erectile dysfunction, it is best to consider placement of a penile prosthesis with simultaneous straightening of the penis. In this circumstance, the prosthesis will support the straightening and allow satisfactory postoperative rigidity for sex.

8. If the penis has a 70-degree bend upward and grafting surgery is performed to correct this condition, what would be the expected result?

The best-case scenario would be satisfactory functional straightening of the penis to less than 20 degrees of curvature along with preservation of sensation, length, and erectile capacity. In men who have good erections preoperatively, 95 percent can expect this type of result. In men who have borderline erections, upwards of 30 percent will have worsening of their erectile capacity after a grafting procedure. The overall worst-case scenario in a man with severe curvature would be inadequate straightening and correction of girth, shortening, loss of sensation, and erectile dysfunction. Thankfully, this worst case scenario is very rare as patients are selected very carefully for this operation.

9. Are there any surgeries for curvature that correct the shape of the penis in the flaccid as well as the erect state?

The surgeries are designed to correct the erect deformity. Irregularities in the flaccid condition are not felt to be clinically significant and may not be correctable as the tissues are soft and naturally take on different shapes. All men have some irregularities in the shape of the penis such as draping to one side or another or even kinked a bit. The key is that when the penis is erect, that it is functionally straight enough to allow penetrative sexual activity. You should also be aware that no man has a perfectly straight penis. Experts believe that curvature in any direction up to 30 degrees will typically not interfere with sex.

10. Once I have surgery, what is the risk of having incomplete straightening?

Your risk of having incomplete straightening following straightening surgery is low. Reports on patients who have undergone straightening operations with up to five years of follow-up show that the rate of incomplete straightening is in the 1 to 5 percent range.

11. How likely is it that if I undergo successful penile straightening by plication or grafting, I will have a recurrence at a later time?

Only recently have studies begun to look at long-term results. For the most part, the published literature on surgery shows a recurrence rate in the 1-10 percent range over the first five years after surgery. It is not clear whether this is due to a new injury or if there is further scarring in the initial area of the plaque. The highest rates of recurrence are reported with the Nesbit plication procedure, where a segment of tissue has been excised. It may be that there is a separation of the repair, resulting in recurrence or that there is a tear/disruption of the sutures. Other investigators have noted that, following the plication operation, sutures are more likely to tear out or break with a strong erection or during intercourse resulting in recurrence.

Note: In my experience with the plication technique where there is no excision of tissue, my recurrence rate with up to seven-year follow-up is approximately 1 percent. It appears that the very great majority of men who undergo any type of plication operation have a very high rate of sustained straightness.

For men who have undergone incision or partial excision and grafting, recurrence rates are similarly low. As of the current time there does not appear to be a greater likelihood of recurrent curvature with any of the grafts except with tunica vaginalis grafts where up to 50 percent of patients have been reported to develop scarring of the graft, resulting in recurrent curvature.

A recent nonpublished report with a small series of patients undergoing grafting with SIS (small intestinal submucosa) grafts has also shown a high rate of recurrence, in the 50 percent range. The reports using the more commonly employed "off-the-shelf" grafts of pericardium, *fascia lata*, and dermis have shown recurrent curvature in less than 5 percent of patients up to five years after surgery. The examination of long-term results following any grafting procedure is now under review in many centers.

One concern is whether the grafting operation is more apt to result in recurrent curvature, diminished sensitivity, and progressive loss of erectile rigidity over time. Due to the recognized complexity of this operation and the potential for more profound side effects due to this complexity, it is, again, only recommended that a grafting procedure be performed when the curvature is extreme (greater than 60 to 70 degrees), when there is significant shortening, or when there is dramatic indentation resulting in a hinge-effect or buckling. The other requirement for proceeding with a grafting procedure is that the patient should have very good-to-excellent-quality erections preoperatively, indicating there is likely little underlying vascular disease before surgery. If there is some erectile dysfunction preoperatively, ED after surgery is more likely.

12. Is surgery the only way to treat chordee or congenital penile curvature?

Currently, there are no medical treatments that can correct this type of penile deformity. The only available treatment for this type of deformity is surgical straightening. It is a simple outpatient surgery using the plication techniques that are also used for Peyronie's disease. In fact, the Nesbit procedure, or variants of this approach, which is now used frequently around the world for Peyronie's disease, was first described in 1965 for the treatment of young boys with chordee.

Resources

American Urological Association (AUA)

1000 Corporate Boulevard
Linthicum, MD 21090
866-746-4282
www.urologyhealth.org

The American Urological Association Foundation was created to provide patient education, to support research, and to improve the treatment, prevention, and cure of urological diseases and conditions. The AUA Web site is written and reviewed by urology experts and features information on Peyronie's disease, including symptoms, causes, getting a diagnosis, treatment options and more. Also available on the site are illustrations, information on clinical trials, and a feature that lets you find a urologist in your area.

Association of Peyronie's Disease Advocates (APDA)

www.peyroniesassociation.org

This association provides information, support, and referral sources for men with Peyronie's disease and their families. APDA also fosters and supports research on the disease to help find treatments and a cure for the disease. The APDA Web site includes an "Ask the Doctor" forum where you can ask questions about Peyronie's disease and receive an answer from a doctor who is an expert in PD. It also provides information on how to choose a doctor to treat Peyronie's disease and offers a locator service to help you find a doctor in your area.

Peyronies.org

2601 West Alameda Avenue, Suite 416
Burbank, California 91505
818-843-1700
www.peyronies.org

Sponsored by a physician who has substantial experience in treating Peyronie's disease, Peyronies.org is a source for patient information. Included in the site are overviews of the disease, its causes, and the treatments currently available. You can also find basic information on the male anatomy and on erections. There is also an anonymous public forum where you can ask questions that will be answered by a doctor.

Sexual Medicine Society of North America

1111 North Plaza Drive, Suite 550
Schaumburg, IL 60173
Phone: 847-517-7225
www.sexhealthmatters.org

Established in 1994 by a group of physicians, researchers, physician assistants, and nurses, the Sexual Medicine Society of North America is dedicated to the education, research, and treatment of sexual function and sexual dysfunction. The not-for-profit organization's web site offers a vast amount of information on general sexual health issues. Although it doesn't include much specifically on Peyronie's disease, it does cover erectile dysfunction, ejaculation problems, and other issues that can be associated with PD. The site also provides a comprehensive list of doctors who provide treatment for sexual dysfunction.

MayoClinic.com

200 First Street SW
Rochester, MN 55905
507-284-2511
www.mayoclinic.com

The Mayo Clinic is the world's first and largest not-for-profit group medical practice. The clinic's Web site, MayoClinic.com, is a reliable source of information on a variety of diseases and medical conditions. The information on Peyronie's disease includes sections on symptoms, causes, risk factors, screening and diagnosis, complications, treatment, prevention, and coping skills.

Glossary

Alprostadil: a drug that causes blood vessel dilation and is used to treat erectile dysfunction.

Atrophy: the wasting away of body tissue.

Autoimmune: a response of one's own body against something in the body.

Benign fibrosis: a noncancerous scarring process.

Cavernosal tissue: spongy, vascular tissue within the penis that fills with blood and expands the outer jacket tissue known as the tunica albuginea.

Chelation: the act of drawing substances out of the body through urination or defecation.

Chordee: congenital curvature of the penis.

Collagenase: an enzyme that breaks down scar tissue.

Combination therapy: the combination of various treatment methods.

Controlled trials: studies in which a placebo is used in comparison to a new drug.

Corpora cavernosa: paired erectile cylinders in the penis.

Glossary

Cystoscope: an instrument used to view the urethra and bladder.

Cystoscopy: a procedure performed to view the interior of the bladder.

Cytokines: chemicals found within scar tissue which can activate and cause ongoing scarring. The most important cytokines stimulating scar formation are TGF-beta (transformation growth factor) and FGF (fibroblast growth factor).

Deformity: an abnormal irregular shape.

Dupuytren's contracture: a condition marked by the shortening of the tendons within the palm of the hand, resulting in the inability to straighten the finger.

Dysmorphic calcification: abnormal bone formation.

Edema: swelling caused by excess fluid in body tissues.

Elastin: a protein that allows tissue to stretch.

Erectile Dysfunction (ED): the term commonly used for impotence or diminished erectile rigidity. Most commonly due to organic and vascular causes but can also be due to psychogenic inhibition.

Excision: the surgical removal of skin or tissue.

Fascia lata: the connective tissue surrounding muscles.

Fibroblasts: cells that make collagen and other components of scar tissue.

Fibrosarcoma: a rare penile cancer.

Fibrosis: scarring that can occur anywhere in the body. Cavernosal fibrosis is a scarring of the spongy, vascular tissue, tunica fibrosis and may be due to trauma or, if excessive, would be consistent with Peyronie's disease.

Flaccid: the soft state of the penis when it is not erect.

Glans: the head of the penis.

Graft: a piece of tissue that is transferred from one place to another and does not contain its own blood supply.

Hinging/hinge-effect: equivalent to buckling, which occurs due to hourglass or substantial indentation resulting in destabilization of the shaft of the penis, which will tend to fold over during penetrative sex.

Hourglass deformity: penile configuration taking on the shape of an hourglass which causes a narrowing of the shaft and may result in a hinge-effect, or buckling, of the penis due to instability most commonly experienced during penetration. The penis will tend to fold or buckle in the area of the hourglass as the column strength of the penis is compromised at the hourglass.

Interferon: a form of a biological modifier, which can change the behavior of the tissues into which it is administered.

Intralesional Injection Therapy: the process of injecting a drug into the scar tissue to change the scar into softer more elastic tissue.

Iontophoresis (EMDA): also known as Electromotive Drug Administration, this is the introduction of a drug through the skin using an electric current.

MUSE (Medicated Urethral System for Erections): a commercial product used as an intraurethral suppository of a drug such as alprostadil. This drug causes blood vessel dialation and is absorbed through the lining of the urethra. A small portion of this drug will move into the erectile tissues causing an erection. MUSE is used primarily for treatment of erectile dysfunction and can be used in patients with Peyronie's disease.

Natural history: the progression of a disease if it is left untreated.

Nitric oxide: a chemical that is released by the penile nerves as a result of sexual stimulation.

Oral erection drugs: agents that are used to stimulate and to improve penile blood flow. These drugs, including Viagra, Levitra, and Cialis, are also known as phosphodiesterase type 5 inhibitors. They block a chemical, found primarily within the penis that breaks down another chemical made by the nerves and blood vessels of the penis in response to sexual stimulation. This chemical, known as cyclic GMP, is necessary for penile vascular dilation. Therefore, these oral erection medications are designed to preserve cyclic GMP and thereby increase penile blood flow, making for better and prolonged erections.

Peyronie's Disease (PD): a scarring disorder involving the tunica albuginea resulting in penile deformity including: curvature, indentation, instability, and shortening. In the early phase, PD can be associated with painful erections and is frequently associated with erectile dysfunction.

Phosphodiesterase (PDE5) inhibitors: oral erection drugs.

Placebo: a nonactive substitute for an active drug. Placebos are frequently used when comparing an active drug in clinical trials to determine its efficacy as compared to a non-active drug.

Plaque: in the context of Peyronie's disease, a plaque is equivalent to a scar. It is not like the plaques found within vascular tissue, which has a substantial cholesterol component.

Plication: bringing together tissue so as to shorten its length. When the tunica albuginea is plicated, typically two incisions are brought together to shorten the side opposite the curvature so as to straighten the penis. There are a variety of ways of accomplishing a plication.

Prosthesis: a device placed within the penis to correct erectile dysfunction.

Radical retropubic prostatectomy: a surgical procedure in which the prostate is removed.

Scrotum: the sac that holds the testicles, epididymes, and associated structures.

Semen: the fluid that carries sperm during ejaculation.

Spontaneous resolution: the act of a disease resolving or going away without treatment.

Temporalis fascia: a thick, flat piece of tissue found under the skin behind the ear.

Tumescent: state of firmness of the penis in which there may be heaviness or extension of the penis, but the penis is not fully erect.

Tunica albuginea: the fibrous multilayered jacket tissue around the cavernosal vascular tissue of the penis. The tunica is naturally thicker on the top, or dorsal, surface of the penis than on the sides, and is thinnest on the undersurface, or ventral, side of the penis.

Tunica vaginalis: a layer of relatively nonelastic tissue surrounding the testicle that can be used in grafting operations.

Urethra: the urinary tube extending from the bladder out to the tip of the penis where the urine and seminal fluid emerge. The urethra does not develop Peyronie's Disease.

Venous leak: a condition in which blood is not being properly trapped and will run out the penis, preventing a full erection. A Peyronie's plaque may alter the function of the venous system which can cause erectile dysfunction in men with Peyronie's disease.

Verapamil: a drug that is a calcium channel blocker that is used in the treatment of Peyronie's disease.

Index

About the Author

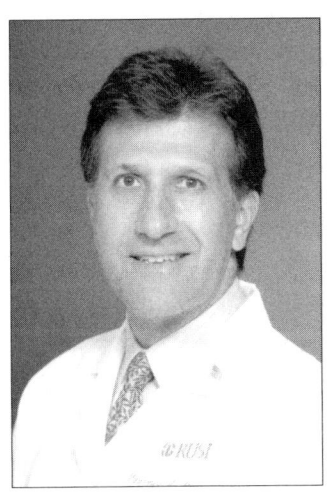

Laurence A. Levine, MD, is Professor in the Department of Urology at Rush University Medical Center in Chicago, Illinois, and Director of the Male Sexual Function and Fertility Program. He is also in group practice with Urology Specialists in Chicago.

Dr. Levine received his medical degree from the University of Colorado Medical School in Denver. He completed an internship and junior residency in general surgery at Tufts–New England Medical Center, a chief residency at the American Hospital of Paris in France, and a residency in urology, Harvard Program, at Brigham and Women's Hospital in Boston, Massachusetts.

Dr. Levine has made a substantial contribution to the medical press in the form of peer-reviewed articles, abstracts, book chapters, and Internet publications regarding Peyronie's disease, male sexual dysfunction, fertility, chronic orchialgia, and reconstructive urology. He is an ad hoc reviewer for *The Journal of Urology, Urology, Journal of Sexual Medicine, Journal of Andrology, Asian Journal of Andrology, British Journal of Urology* and *European Urology*.

Dr. Levine is the editor and contributor to *Peyronie's Disease: A Guide to Clinical Management*, the first textbook on Peyronie's disease, published by Humana Press in 2006. He also has an active involvement in basic science research on Peyronie's disease at Rush University Medical Center where he and his colleagues are looking for the causes and new treatments for this distressing medical problem.

Dr. Levine is a Diplomate of the American Board of Urology. He also served as a member of the AUA Guidelines Panel for the treatment of ED and on the Peyronie's Disease Committee at the World Health Organization First and Second Consultations on Erectile Dysfunction in Paris in 1999 and 2003. He serves on the Board of Directors and is President of the Sexual Medicine Society of North America. He is Past President of the Chicago Urological Society.

For more information about Dr. Levine's urology practice, please visit his Web site: **www.urologyspecialists.net**

1. What inspired you to specialize in urology?

The field of urology offers me the opportunity to work with men and women of all ages. Urology has many different areas of subspecialization such as sexual health, infertility, cancer, stones, and dysfunction involving urination. There are also many fascinating new areas for investigative research. Unlike many specialty areas, urology appears to be expanding rather than contracting.

2. What do you find most rewarding about your work as a urologist?

To me, the most rewarding aspect of being a urologist is having the privilege to care for people suffering from urological disorders and being be able to make a difference in their lives. This may range from such things as eliminating a painful kidney stone, curing cancer, helping an infertile couple have a child, or offering effective therapy for sexual dysfunction and Peyronie's disease.

3.   How did you develop an interest in Peyronie's disease?

During my residency in Boston, I saw very few men with PD. At that time, the only available treatments were Vitamin E, Potaba, and surgery. The oral treatments didn't work and although the surgery was interesting the results were not always satisfying. As a young attending surgeon at the University of Chicago in the late 1980s I continued to see men frustrated and devastated by Peyronie's disease. One day in 1990 while attending a research seminar on wound healing in the hand, verapamil was reported to reduce the production of the primary components of scar. This triggered my interest determining whether verapamil injections into Peyronie's plaques could have a beneficial effect. My first study was presented in 1992 and as a result of the introduction of this new treatment for PD my experience with the disorder expanded rapidly.

4.   Describe the typical male patient who comes to you with PD. What is he feeling and experiencing?

The typical male I see with PD is in his early 50s, but I see men from teenagers to those in their 70s. Usually they don't recall any event where they may have injured their penis. In the acute phase they often notice a pain in the penis with erection, followed by feeling a lump in the penis and then developing a deformity. Many of these men delay evaluation fearing that the lump may be a cancer or hoping that it will simply go away. Unfortunately, many of these men who seek medical care do not obtain proper evaluation as there are many misconceptions about Peyronie's disease held by doctors in general. These men are, typically, psychologically and physically devastated about the change in their penis, and it is a major blow to their manhood. This results in frustration, anger, depression, a feeling of helplessness, and marked diminished self-esteem.

5. With the treatments available today, what percentage of men will see improvement in their condition after treatment?

For men who are either not candidates for surgery, because their disease has not yet stabilized, or are not psychologically ready to accept surgery, there is no non-surgical cure, but there are treatment options which can prevent progression or improve function. At this time, intralesional verapamil injection is the most scientifically sensible approach. In my studies, up to 60 percent of men will see some improvement following a course of verapamil injections. The combination of oral and injection therapy combined with external traction therapy may be the best non-surgical approach today with hopes of encouraging tissue remodeling and correction of deformity.

Surgery remains the most rapid and reliable way to correct penile deformity. Most men I see are not eager to have surgery and clearly the goal is to find a medical treatment which is effective, non-toxic, and easy to administer. The search for such a remedy is ongoing.

6. What is the most common type of treatment that you deliver to patients?

Currently, the majority of my patients receive my three-armed approach, which includes oral treatment with Pentoxifylline and L-arginine, intralesional injection of verapamil, and daily use of the Fastsize penile extender to encourage tissue remodeling. The remaining men undergo surgery with either plication, incision and grafting when the curvature is severe, or placement of a prosthesis when there is preexisting erectile dysfunction.

7. What do you consider the biggest advance in treating PD in the last 10 years?

I believe that the introduction of intralesional verapamil injection was the biggest advance in the treatment of Peyronie's disease as it offers a reasonably effective and safe nonsurgical treatment that was not available before. As a result of clinical studies on verapamil there has been enhanced awareness of this disorder.

8. Describe one recent patient that stands out in your mind. What were his concerns, how was he treated, and what was his response treatment?

Recently, a man came to me with advanced Peyronie's disease. He had seen many physicians and urologists in his home state but without benefit. He told me that he came to Chicago for help, because he was considering suicide if there was no improvement in his condition. He began the three-armed program and noted rapid reduction of his penile pain. Although he has not completed the treatment protocol, he notes improvement in his condition, allowing him to be sexually active again. He is still devastated by the changes in the loss of his penile length, but he is coping better with the change.

Addicus Books Consumer Health Titles

Visit our online catalog at www.AddicusBooks.com

Organizations, associations, corporations, hospitals, and other groups may qualify for special discounts when ordering more than twenty-four copies. For more information, please contact the Special Sales Department at Addicus Books.

Phone (402) 330-7493

Email: info@AddicusBooks.com